Prenatal Drug Exposure: Kinetics and Dynamics

Editors:

C. Nora Chiang, Ph.D.

Charles C. Lee, Ph.D.

Division of Preclinical Research
National Institute on Drug Abuse

NIDA Research Monograph 60
1985

U.S. DEPARTMENT OF HEALTH AND HUMAN SERVICES
Public Health Service
Alcohol, Drug Abuse, and Mental Health Administration

National Institute on Drug Abuse
5600 Fishers Lane
Rockville, Maryland 20857

NIDA Research Monographs are prepared by the research divisions of the National Institute on Drug Abuse and published by its Office of Science. The primary objective of the series is to provide critical reviews of research problem areas and techniques, the content of state-of-the-art conferences, and integrative research reviews. Its dual publication emphasis is rapid and targeted dissemination to the scientific and professional community.

Parklawn Building, 5600 Fishers Lane, Rockville, Maryland 20857

Prenatal Drug Exposure: Kinetics and Dynamics

ACKNOWLEDGMENT

Dr. Charles C. Lee, coeditor of this monograph, was on sabbatical leave from the University of Houston during 1984 and serving as a member of the professional staff with the Division of Preclinical Research, National Institute on Drug Abuse, by an agreement under the Intergovernmental Personnel Act of 1970.

This monograph is based upon papers presented at a technical review on prenatal drug exposure and consequences of maternal drug use which took place on September 24-25, 1984, at Bethesda, Maryland. The meeting was sponsored by the Division of Clinical Research and Division of Preclinical Research, National Institute on Drug Abuse. The clinical papers have been published separately as NIDA Research Monograph 59, Current Research on the Consequences of Maternal Drug Abuse.

DHHS publication number (ADM)85-1413
Printed 1985

NIDA Research Monographs are indexed in the Index Medicus. They are selectively included in the coverage of American Statistics Index, BioSciences Information Service, Chemical Abstracts, Current Contents, Psychological Abstracts, and Psychopharmacology Abstracts.

Contents

Contents

Introduction and Overview

C. Nora Chiang and Charles C. Lee

It has become obvious from both animal experiments and clinical observations that the placenta does not act as a barrier to protect the fetus from exposure to xenobiotics taken by the mother. Nearly all drugs or foreign chemicals, following maternal exposure, enter the fetus and may exert adverse effects, depending on the reactivity (dynamics) of the drug in the fetus and the extent of fetal drug exposure, which may be assessed from the kinetics of the drug in the maternal-fetal unit. The fetus may be affected through the direct action of a drug as well as indirectly due to drug effects on the mother. Hence, it is a primary health concern to understand the adverse effects of a drug, taken by the mother, on the fetus. In addition, it is of paramount importance to determine the kinetics and the dynamics of a drug in the maternal-fetal unit in order to elucidate the mechanisms of drug action.

Studies in humans regarding drug effects due to prenatal exposure are usually limited because of ethical and technical considerations. Such studies are usually restricted to clinical observations of pregnancy outcomes or the determination of drug concentrations in maternal and fetal biological fluid samples collected at the time of delivery. Much of the research assessing the potentially harmful effects of prenatal drug exposure, and particularly the mechanisms of such effects, is performed in animals. Because of the continuous morphological and physiological alterations during pregnancy in the mother, placenta, and fetus, both the kinetics and dynamics of a drug in the maternal-fetal unit may change progressively. Studies on the effects and mechanisms of drug action in the fetus are therefore very complicated and involve a diverse range of disciplines. Furthermore, there are questions concerning the extrapolation of animal data to humans since there are anatomical differences in the structure of placenta and species differences in the pharmacologic action (dynamics) and the disposition (kinetics) of a drug.

The experimental complexity and broad spectrum of prenatal pharmacology and toxicology require the exchange of information as well as integrated efforts among scientists from different disciplines, including clinical research, chemistry, biochemistry, pharmacokinetics, pharmacology, and physiology. To coordinate an effort for information exchange and interdisciplinary interaction, the National Institute on Drug Abuse sponsored a technical review on September 24 and 25, 1984. This volume presents the proceedings of the preclinical portion of the technical review. It focuses primarily on the current research findings of prenatal drug effects and current approaches for the investigation of mechanisms of prenatal drug effects through applications of state-of-the-art technology. In addition, an appendix containing a comprehensive review of literature data regarding the dynamics and kinetics of drugs in the maternal-fetal unit has been added as a supplement. Research articles presented of the clinical portion of the meeting are collected in a separate volume entitled "Current Research on the Consequences of Maternal Drug Abuse."

Various animal preparations have been used for the investigation of prenatal drug effects. An overview of animal models was presented by Dr. Rudolph. The presentation highlighted the pregnant ewe as an animal model for quantitative assessment of the extent of drug exposure and the intensity of pharmacological/physiological responses of the fetus. Techniques for the preparation of the pregnant ewe for such investigations were illustrated. This preparation is highly praised and indeed provides a useful model for studies of drug effects in the fetus. Nevertheless, an extrapolation to the human situation must be made with caution.

Drug disposition plays an important role in the elicitation or termination of a pharmacologic effect. The biotransformation of drugs or other exogenous chemicals in the placental-fetal unit was presented by Dr. Juchau. Recent findings indicate that fetal liver and placenta of human and nonhuman primates develop drug-metabolizing enzyme activities during gestational maturation, while other subprimate animals in general lack enzyme activities at this stage. One set of drug-metabolizing enzymes (monooxygenases) in the placenta has been found to exhibit increased activity in tobacco smokers. Preliminary evidence suggests that these enzymes may catalyze the generation of highly reactive metabolic intermediates capable of eliciting deleterious effects in the fetus and newborn. Since research in this area is still in a developmental stage, continuing efforts are required to establish the toxicological or pharmacological significance of these drug-metabolizing enzymes.

The application of pharmacokinetics, a quantitative description of the time course of a drug in the body, to studies of drug transport mechanisms between the mother and fetus and the elicited pharmacological effects was discussed by Dr. Benet. Using the ewe model, pharmacokinetic principles were demonstrated with acetaminophen as a model drug for studies of the transfer of drug and metabolites between the mother and fetus as well as fetal disposition of all chemical entities. Pharmacokinetics, as applied in drug abuse research, will certainly help to provide insight into the extent of fetal exposure and toxic consequences.

Prenatal effects of diazepam on rodents were discussed by Dr. Miller. Reports indicate that persistent and selective alteration of the central nervous system is induced in rats following low-dose diazepam exposure during the last week of gestation and that coadministration of a diazepam antagonist effectively prevents these alterations. The data suggest that administration of diazepam during pregnancy may result in permanent, selective, receptor-mediated alterations in behavioral and transmitter functions in the neonate.

The overall opiate effects on the somatic and neurobiological development of the fetus and/or the infant were summarized by Dr. Zagon. Laboratory investigations revealed that the actions of opiate agonists were stereospecific and subject to blockade by coadministration of opiate antagonists. This suggests that the locus of opiate action is at the level of the opiate receptor. Recent research findings, which suggest that opioid antagonists affect fetal development, led to the speculation that endogenous opioid peptides may serve to regulate growth through interaction with opiate receptors. The role of endogenous opioids on fetal development clearly needs further investigation.

The adverse effects of opioids on the offspring due to maternal drug exposure have been well documented, although the mechanisms of action are not clear. In utero monitoring, utilizing the pregnant ewe model, of the direct effects of morphine exposure on fetal behavioral, respiratory, and cardiovascular functions was presented by Dr. Szeto. Results showed that morphine exhibited a biphasic dose-response relationship, excitation at low dose and suppression at high dose, and the fetal narcotic abstinence symptom was precipitated in utero after a short 2-hour low-dose morphine exposure. These findings suggest that the fetus may undergo a cycle of acute physical dependence and withdrawal when opiates are administered to normal clinical patients. Further research in this area is needed to provide further insight into mechanisms for the neurobehavioral disturbances observed in children born to pregnant narcotic users.

Noninvasive methods are clearly preferable for the study of drug distribution in maternal and fetal tissues. The use of the new and noninvasive technique, Positron Emission Tomography (PET) for the study of morphine and heroin distribution in pregnant monkeys was illustrated by Dr. Lindberg. Following drug administration, both drugs readily distribute to the fetus, with heroin reaching the fetus more rapidly than morphine. In combination with pharmacokinetic modeling, PET may prove to be a powerful tool for the evaluation of rapid distribution and disposition of drugs in the maternal-fetal unit. It is also a potentially useful means for the determination of specific sites of drug action in the fetus.

Clinical reports on infants born to tobacco-smoking mothers suggest several adverse effects. According to Dr. Kuhnert, three components of cigarette smoke--cadmium, lead, and thiocyanate--were present at substantially higher than normal concentrations in the newborn of cigarette smokers. These components were shown to exhibit some deleterious biological activities. For example, cadmium was shown to be placental-toxic in both animal studies and in the in vitro human placenta preparation, as presented by Dr. Miller. The factors that clinically affect the infant or fetus are not yet identified. Dr. Kuhnert also reported adverse effects for infants born to mothers who used phencyclidine, meperidine, or alcohol during pregnancy. Quantitative analysis of these drugs in the biological fluids of infants at birth demonstrated their presence.

All data gathered to date support the notion that nearly all drugs taken by the pregnant mother readily cross the placenta to the fetus. Research efforts to determine the concentrations of drugs/chemicals in body fluids of the newborn of maternal drug users have provided valuable information for the assessment of potential adverse effects to the infants. These efforts should be continued with particular emphasis on the application of new analytical technologies which enable drug determination in microliter volumes of sample fluid.

It is well recognized that information on perinatal effect of drugs of abuse is very limited. In many instances, the available data are confusing or contradictory. Discrepancies may be attributed to different methodologies employed, different animal species studied, and varying routes of drug administration, doses, and dosage forms. Despite the limitations of the animal model, it is generally agreed that animal studies do provide valuable information on prenatal drug effects. It is recommended, however, that researchers be cautious about the selection of the animal model as well as the route, dose, and dosage form of the drug to be administered. It is further emphasized that a dose-response curve should be generated for the selection of a proper dose for the animal studies, as some drugs may exert multiphasic pharmacological effects.

In summary, it is clear that further research efforts are needed in this critical area to further contribute to the substantial base of knowledge on prenatal drug effects due to maternal drug exposure which has been generated over years of research. As new technologies advance, more sophisticated means for the investigation of the mechanisms of drug action can be implemented. Of particular importance is integrated research involving interdisciplinary collaboration which will certainly contribute to the overall understanding of the preclinical and clinical facets of the subject. Combining clinical and laboratory findings can be anticipated to yield an improved basis for the prediction and minimization of toxicities in humans through more effective treatment and prevention efforts on the part of both physicians and the lay public.

AUTHORS

C. Nora Chiang, Ph.D.
Division of Preclinical Research
National Institute on Drug Abuse
5600 Fishers Lane
Rockville, Maryland 20857

Charles C. Lee, Ph.D.
University of Houston
Texas Medical Center
1441 Moursund Ave.
Houston, Texas 77030

Animal Models for Study of Fetal Drug Exposure

Abraham M. Rudolph

Increasing concerns have developed regarding the potential harmful effects on fetal development of drugs injected into or ingested by the mother, and from her exposure to chemicals encountered in occupations or the environment. Much of the earlier work regarding these potential hazards was done in humans, and involved the detection of drugs or their metabolites in umbilical cord blood at the time of delivery, or in urine in the newborn infant soon after birth. Although detection of the parent drug reflected passage across the placenta, the presence of metabolites did not confirm that the drug itself was transferred, because the placenta may have been permeable to the metabolite but not to the drug itself. Additional earlier studies in the human were concerned with the effects that drugs taken by the mother had on fetal function. Moya and Thorndike (1962) reviewed the work done on detection of drugs in umbilical cord blood, and on observation of behavior and certain physiological parameters of the human infant after birth.

Another major interest in drug effects on the fetus concerned the examination of their teratogenic effects. Considerable attention has been directed toward studying the potential of drugs administered to the mother at different stages of embryonic and fetal development to induce congenital defects or even embryonic or fetal death. Most of this work has been done in small rodents (Warkany and Takacs 1959). In addition, much knowledge has been derived from examination of the coincidental occurrence of specific congenital defects and administration of certain drugs to the human mother.

More recently, interest has been directed toward obtaining more specific information about factors that influence drug transfer across the placenta and drug distribution in the fetus, and about the effects of drugs on fetal physiological and biochemical functions. The perfused human placenta in vitro has been used extensively to examine transfer of metabolites and drugs (Schneider et al. 1972). There are several major concerns regarding these studies. First, the perfusion medium has usually been an electrolyte solution, sometimes with low molecular weight dextran; the flow rates are usually quite low compared with what might be expected in vivo, raising questions about the degree of vasoconstriction present. Also, the duration of viability of the preparation has not been established.

Physiological responses of the human fetus to drugs have been difficult to assess. Heart rate responses can be monitored, and Schifferli and Caldeyro-Barcia (1973) studied effects on fetal heart rate after administering atropine or beta-adrenergic drugs to the mother. Recently, it has also become possible to monitor human fetal respiratory movements by ultrasound techniques, and it will be possible to examine the effects of drugs on this activity.

In this presentation, I will not address the use of animal models for assessing the teratogenic effects of drugs. I plan to discuss some models that have been used, and some that have the potential to be used for studying pharmacokinetics and pharmacodynamics in the fetal placental unit, and to address some of the limitations of these studies. The following issues will be considered, along with models available for their study:

1. Placental transfer of drugs and their metabolites;
2. Fetal distribution;
3. Intrauterine distribution and excretion of drugs and metabolites;
4. Fetal drug metabolism;
5. Pharmacological effects of drugs and metabolites.

PLACENTAL TRANSFER

The influence of physical properties on the diffusibility of substances across the placenta has been reviewed by Faber (1973). Lipid soluble materials diffuse readily across the placenta. Rate of movement is largely affected by umbilical and uterine blood flow rates rather than by permeability, because this determines the rate of delivery and removal of the substance at the exchange site. However, transfer of lipid insoluble substances is dependent on molecular size and on the morphology of the placental membrane. The rate of transfer of lipid insoluble substances is proportional to their coefficient of free diffusion in water. If molecular size is very large, there may be no diffusion. Since placental morphology is very different in different species, pore size will be quite variable, and diffusibility is markedly affected. Thus, the rabbit and guinea pig have a hemoendothelial placenta: the fetal and maternal blood streams are separated only by fetal endothelium. Because of this, molecules larger than plasma albumin can diffuse across the placenta. The sheep placenta is syndesmochorial; it has five layers separating fetal and maternal blood: maternal endothelium and connective tissue, and fetal trophoblast, connective tissue, and endothelium. The placentae of the human and the primate are hemochorial, consisting of three fetal layers. Thus, because of the histology of the membrane, the sheep placenta presents a considerably greater diffusion barrier than the human placenta, which in turn is less permeable than the rabbit or guinea pig placenta. These potentially enormous differences in placental diffusing capacity must be appreciated in experimental studies of drug transfer.

Diffusion rate is dependent on the mean concentration difference between maternal and fetal blood. As Faber points out, the relevant concentrations are those of physically dissolved material, not the total content. Thus, protein binding of drugs will have a marked effect on placental transfer, either from mother to fetus, or fetus to mother. Potentially, fetal and maternal protein-binding capacities may be different, apart from the fact that, at least in some species, albumin concentrations are lower in fetal blood.

Several animal models have been used to study drug transfer across the placenta. Mirkin (1973) described a technique for examining transfer and tissue distribution of a drug in the fetus by injection of an isotopically labeled drug into the mother. After killing the animals at various intervals after injection, whole fetuses were examined by radioautography. Although this technique does demonstrate which fetal tissues are labeled, there are several drawbacks. First, only small rodents can be used; second, caution would have to be exercised that the tissue labelling was not caused by passage of labeled metabolites rather than the parent drug; and third, the technique does not provide quantitative data regarding drug transfer.

Several investigators have used techniques for studying drug transfer to and from the fetus by placing intravascular catheters in the fetus and mother, and administering drugs either to the fetus or mother. Maternal and fetal plasma concentrations were measured either after a bolus injection or after infusion. Many of these studies were done acutely in anesthetized animals; this raises serious concerns regarding the reliability of any quantitative measurements of transfer rates because anesthesia or acute stress could greatly modify circulatory dynamics in both mother and fetus and also influence hormonal and metabolic activity. Fouron (1973) studied placental transfer of digoxin in the dog acutely under anesthesia after either acute or chronic administration of the drug. Cosmi (1976) studied transfer of anesthetic agents and other drugs in sheep; and Ruckebusch et al. (1976) reported on the transfer of thiopental, meperidine, and acepromazine (a phenothiazine) in sheep, as well as monitoring some fetal responses to these drugs. Also, Szeto et al. (1978) studied some aspects of pharmacokinetics of meperidine in the fetus and mother in a chronically catheterized pregnant sheep model.

Numerous studies of similar type have been performed in chronically catheterized fetal and maternal sheep, in which a fetal hindlimb artery and vein and maternal artery and vein have been catheterized. This model is useful for determining the rapidity of transfer of drugs in either direction across the placenta and the relative fetal and maternal plasma concentrations. Thus, Morishima et al. (1972, 1975) showed that lidocaine, when injected into the mother, appears in fetal plasma very quickly. With this model, it is also possible, after a bolus of the drug is injected into the fetal or maternal circulation, to determine its biological half-life in the fetus or mother, as well as the presence of, and rates of disappearance of, metabolites. However, the information derived does not differentiate between actual placental transfer and removal by metabolism or excretion by other routes.

Transfer rates of drugs across the placenta can be measured more specifically by application of the Fick principle. Meschia et al. (1966) first applied this approach to measure umbilical and uterine blood flows in pregnant sheep by infusing antipyrine into the fetus. The rate of removal of drug to the uterus and its contents is measured by the equation

$$\dot{A} = \dot{Q}_{ut} \times (C_{uta} - C_{utv})$$

where $\dot{A}$ is amount removed, $\dot{Q}_{ut}$ is uterine blood flow, and C_{uta} and C_{utv} are concentrations of drug in uterine artery and vein at steady state. This technique has limitations because the sheep uterus has several draining veins, and sampling from a single vein may not be representative of mixed uterine venous blood. Also, uterine venous blood is a mixture of blood derived from placental site perfusion as well as uterine musculature. Myometrial blood flow in the sheep in mid- to late-gestation accounts for only about 15% of total uterine blood flow, but this must be considered in estimates of placental transfer.

The amount of a drug that is removed or taken up at the placenta on the fetal side can be calculated similarly from the equation

$$\dot{A} = \dot{Q}_{um} \times (C_{umv} - C_{uma})$$

where $\dot{Q}_{um}$ is umbilical blood flow and C_{umv} and C_{uma} are concentrations of drug in umbilical vein and artery, respectively, at steady state. Problems with umbilical venous sampling may present difficulties in making accurate measurements. A technique used commonly to catheterize the umbilical vein is to pass a catheter from a peripheral cotyledonary vein centrally into one of the two main veins (Rudolph and Heymann 1980). It is possible that the sample obtained may not reflect mixed umbilical venous blood. To overcome this, we developed a method for chronically catheterizing the common intra-abdominal segment of the umbilical vein (Young et al. 1974), but recent experience has shown that there is no significant difference in concentrations in the common vein as compared with the two main veins.

Uterine and umbilical blood flow can be measured by several techniques. The antipyrine steady-state diffusion method mentioned above suffers from the inability to make repeated measurements after any manipulation without waiting a considerable period for a new steady state to be achieved. Techniques for applying electromagnetic flow transducers to the vessels have been described for both the mother and fetus. Flow transducers can be applied to the branches of the uterine artery, but to measure total flow, the transducer can be applied to the distal aorta beyond the origins of the common iliac arteries. In the sheep, this segment of the aorta gives rise to the two uterine arteries, from which also arise some small branches to the pelvis. Thus, measurement of flow at this site slightly overestimates the uterine blood flow. In the fetal lamb, we demonstrated that the umbilical arteries arise from a short distal segment beyond the common iliac artery origin. We have described the technique for applying a flow transducer to this segment to measure total umbilical blood flow (Berman et al. 1975). Because some small arteries arising from the umbilical arteries supply pelvic tissue, the measured flow slightly overestimates actual umbilical blood flow. The great advantage of this technique is that blood flow can be measured instantaneously and rapid alterations can be monitored.

The radionuclide-labeled microsphere technique is a useful method for measuring both umbilical and uterine blood flows (Rudolph and Heymann 1967; Heymann et al. 1977). In the mother, a catheter must be introduced retrograde through a peripheral artery and advanced to the left ventricle. If the placental portion of the uterus is separated from the surrounding myometrium at autopsy, it is possible to measure uterine blood flow to each portion separately. In the fetus, the microspheres can be injected into a peripheral vein while a reference sample is collected from the descending aorta or one of its branches. It is also feasible to measure umbilical blood flow to the placental cotyledons separate from the amniotic and chorionic membranes.

The placenta has high metabolic activity and a fairly large volume. Drugs delivered to the placental site either from the maternal or fetal circulations will be distributed in the placental volume. Also, some of the drug may be metabolized by the placenta. Thus, even at steady state, the calculated uptake of drug by the placenta on the fetal side may not equal the calculated amount leaving the uterine circulation at the placental site. The difference is a reflection of placental removal of drug.

It should also be appreciated that the uptake or release calculated from the Fick equations above represents net transfer. Some of the drug in the umbilical artery may cross to the maternal circulation, whereas some in the uterine artery may enter the fetal circulation.

FETAL DISTRIBUTION AND EXCRETION OF DRUGS AND METABOLITES

The fetal circulation is characterized by the presence of shunts which provide preferential distribution of oxygen and substrates to upper body organs, and also function as a partial bypass of the lungs. The radioautography studies developed by Mirkin (1973) are not quantitative enough to define distribution patterns of drugs in fetal tissues. The blood flow patterns in the fetus are important to our understanding of how drugs and chemicals delivered to the fetus across the placenta into umbilical venous blood are distributed in the fetus. It is also important in experimental studies in which drugs are infused directly into the fetus for pharmacokinetic or pharmacodynamic studies. Furthermore, because of the shunting, arterial concentrations of drugs may be very different in upper and lower body arteries.

The patterns of blood flow in major venous channels have been studied in fetal lambs by applying the radionuclide-labeled microsphere technique. Simultaneous injection of microspheres into various peripheral veins has defined the flow patterns shown in figure 1. Umbilical venous blood contributes about 40% of total venous return; about 55% normally passes through the ductus venosus, thus bypassing the liver, while the remainder is distributed to the left and right lobes of the liver. Portal venous blood is distributed exclusively to the right lobe of the liver (Edelstone et al. 1978). Distal inferior vena caval blood is joined by blood from the left and right hepatic veins and the ductus venosus just below the diaphragm. However, blood does not mix completely in the thoracic portion of the inferior vena cava. We have shown that ductus venosus blood streams preferentially through the foramen ovale to the left atrium, whereas distal inferior vena caval blood preferentially flows through the tricuspid valve into the right ventricle (Reuss and Rudolph 1980; Edelstone and Rudolph 1979). Superior vena caval blood passes almost exclusively through the tricuspid valve into the right ventricle. Right ventricular blood largely flows through the ductus arteriosus to the descending aorta, while left ventricular blood is ejected into the ascending aorta. These flow patterns account for the higher oxygen saturation in ascending aortic blood as compared with descending aortic blood in the fetus, and also could result in higher concentrations of drugs in ascending aortic blood when they enter the fetus through the placenta.

We have also shown that left hepatic venous blood follows the preferential streaming pattern of ductus venosus blood, whereas right hepatic venous blood is distributed in a similar manner to distal inferior vena caval blood.

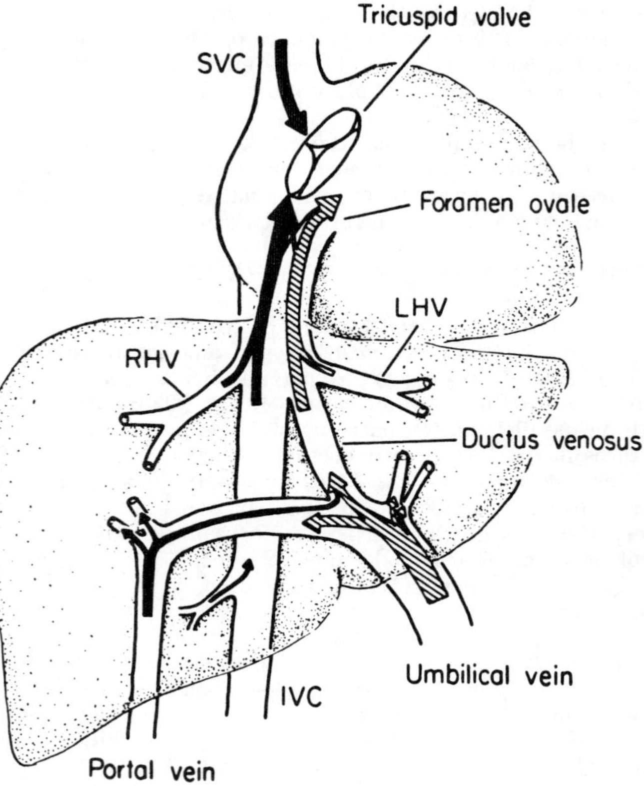

FIGURE 1. The course and distribution of venous blood entering the heart in the fetus is depicted. Umbilical venous blood enters the hepatic hilum and gives off branches to the left lobe. The ductus venosus carries predominantly umbilical venous blood driectly to the inferior vena cava. The umbilical vein then arches to the right to join the portal vein. Almost all portal venous blood enters the right lobe of the liver. The right hepatic venous blood joins the abdominal inferior vena caval stream to be preferentially distributed through the tricuspid valve. Left hepatic venous blood joins the ductus venosus stream and these two well-oxygenated bloods are preferentially directed through the foramen ovale. The superior vena caval blood is almost completely directed through the tricuspid valve (From Rudolph 1983, copyright 1983, American Association for the Study of Liver Diseases.)

These distribution patterns could greatly influence concentrations of drugs reaching different organs, depending on their route of administration and on the rate of metabolism in various organs. Thus, if a drug enters the umbilical circulation it first reaches the fetal liver, but about half passes directly through the ductus venosus. If the drug is rapidly metabolized by the liver, up to half of that entering the fetus may be removed on the first pass. If the drug is administered through the portal vein, it will reach the right lobe of the liver in highest concentration, with much lower concentrations reaching the left lobe of the liver. When a drug is infused into a forelimb vein, it will not be distributed to the brain or heart on the first pass, and if the drug is readily removed by the placenta, large amounts may be necessary to have an effect on the heart or brain. In the same fetus, drugs infused at the same ratio could thus exert very different effects, depending on the route of administration.

INTRAUTERINE DISTRIBUTION AND EXCRETION

In addition to distribution of drug administered to the mother into the fetal body, some drugs may enter the chorioallantoic membranes and amniotic and allantoic sacs. Exchanges between allantoic and amniotic fluids and the fetal or maternal circulations are not clearly established. The amniotic fluid surrounds the fetus, but the allantoic sac occupies a small segment of the uterine space. In the latter trimester of the sheep, the allantoic space is well defined in the horn of the uterus and in the cervical region, but in the body of the uterus the allantoic and amniotic membranes are closely applied and there is little allantoic cavity in this region (Mellor 1980). Because of this, there could well be poor mixing within the allantoic cavity. Similarly, although the fetus is surrounded by amniotic fluid, the degree of mixing of substances that enter the amniotic fluid is not well established. In early gestation in the sheep, the fluid is a clear liquid and mixing may be good, but beyond about 120 days gestation the fluid becomes increasingly viscid and considerable mucus is present, and distribution of materials added to it may be quite poor.

It is possible to place catheters into the amniotic and allantoic sacs and to maintain them chronically. The amniotic catheter can be readily inserted adjacent to the fetal body. To catheterize the allantoic sac, the muscle of the horn of the uterus is carefully incised and the allantoic cavity is entered; it is recognized by the presence of clear yellowish fluid, in contrast with amniotic fluid, which is often turbid and, in later gestation, viscid. Also, the cotyledonary branches of the umbilical arteries and veins are clearly visible on the chorionic membrane.

The allantoic and amniotic spaces may have a prominent role in kinetics of the parent drug or its metabolites. If the drug or metabolite enters these spaces, it could be reabsorbed into the maternal or fetal circulation. The drug or metabolite may enter the amniotic sac from fetal urinary output via the urethra, or the allantoic sac from urine via the urachus. In addition, drugs may enter the amniotic fluid in tracheal fluid, secreted by the lung, or possibly via the gastrointestinal tract, but the latter source is not likely.

The excretion of drug or metabolites by the fetal kidney can be measured readily in the lamb fetus in which a catheter is implanted chronically into the bladder. This can be done directly through a suprapubic abdominal incision (Iwamoto and Rudolph 1983), but can also be readily accomplished by passing a catheter through the urachus either intra-abdominally or as it enters the umbilical cord, external to the umbilical ring. I now prefer the urachus approach because, since the urachus is ligated, urine will not enter the allantoic sac. Also, to be sure that no urine enters the amniotic sac, the urethra can be ligated at the skin surface. If this is done, the urinary catheter must be allowed to drain, so that retention does not occur. When catheters are placed in the bladder and in the allantoic and amniotic sacs, it is possible to measure the urinary excretion rates of drugs and their metabolites, and also examine their rates of entry and removal from the allantoic and amniotic fluid. As mentioned above, because there may be problems of even distribution of substances in the allantoic and amniotic fluid, the information regarding drug and metabolite concentrations and kinetics in the allantoic and amniotic sacs may not be precise.

FETAL DRUG METABOLISM

A great deal of work has been done on developmental aspects of enzymes involved in drug metabolism, but most studies have concentrated on detection of enzymatic activity in vitro in microsomal fractions or homogenates of fetal organs, or in fetal cell cultures. This work has been reviewed extensively by Dutton (1978). However, the techniques used may possibly interfere with activity of some enzymes and, furthermore, may activate an enzyme present in inactive form, but which may not be active in vivo. Study of metabolism of drugs by the fetus in vivo have taken two directions. First, analysis of metabolites of the drug in fetal blood provide an indication that the fetus has the capacity to metabolize the drug, assuming that the metabolites do not cross the placenta. If they do cross the placenta, it is difficult to determine whether they are derived from maternal metabolism. Also, measurement of metabolite concentration does not indicate where the drug is being metabolized.

We have developed a preparation in fetal lambs which allows the direct measurement of rates of metabolism by the liver. Catheters are implanted into a lower limb artery and vein, an umbilical vein, a mesenteric venous tributary of the portal vein, and a left or right hepatic vein. These techniques have been reported previously (Bristow et al. 1981). Blood flow to each lobe of the liver from the umbilical veins, to the portal vein, and to the hepatic artery can be measured using the radionuclide-labeled microsphere method. By measuring concentrations of drugs or metabolites in the various vessels and using the blood flow data, rates of hepatic uptake or release can be calculated by the Fick method. We have shown that, in the fetus, only a very small percentage of liver blood supply is derived from the hepatic artery, and it can readily be discounted in these calculations. Thus, for the left lobe

$$\dot{A} = \dot{Q}_{Luv} \times C_{uv} - \dot{Q}_{Luv} \times C_{Lhv}$$

and for the right lobe

$$\dot{A} = (\dot{Q}_{Ruv} \times C_{uv} + \dot{Q}_{Rpv} \times C_{pv}) - (\dot{Q}_{Ruv} + \dot{Q}_{Rpv}) \times C_{Rhv}$$

Where $\dot{A}$ is the amount taken up or released, $\dot{Q}_{Luv}$ is blood flow to the left liver lobe from umbilical vein, and C_{uv} and C_{Lhv} are concentrations of drug or metabolites in umbilical venous and left hepatic venous blood.

$\dot{Q}_{Ruv}$ and $\dot{Q}_{Rpv}$ are blood flows to the right liver lobe from the umbilical and portal veins. C_{uv}, C_{pv}, and C_{Rhv} are concentrations in umbilical vein, portal vein, and right hepatic vein.

These calculations depend for reliability on adequate concentration differences across the liver; if this does not occur, it may be necessary to use radioisotopically labeled drugs, with measurement of specific activity of metabolites in hepatic venous blood.

Recently, we have also developed a preparation in fetal lambs in which the renal vein is catheterized chronically (Iwamoto and Rudolph 1983). In association with lower limb artery catheterization and measurement of renal blood flow either by the microsphere method or by clearance techniques, the rate of uptake of drugs or release of metabolites from the kidney can be calculated.

PHARMACOLOGICAL EFFECTS OF DRUGS AND METABOLITES

Numerous fetal physiological and biochemical functions can now be monitored in the chronically instrumented fetal lamb. Heart rate and arterial pressure can be monitored from intra-arterial catheters, or heart rate and electrocardiogram can be recorded from chronically implanted ECG leads sewn to fetal skin. Venous pressures or atrial and ventricular pressures can be recorded from catheters inserted directly, or via peripheral vessels.

Continuous measurement of blood flow in several fetal vessels has been achieved by chronic implantation of electromagnetic flow transducers around the vessel. Thus, umbilical blood flow can be measured by placing a flow transducer around the common umbilical artery (Berman et al. 1975) or the common umbilical vein (Oakes et al. 1976). Transducers around the pulmonary trunk measure right ventricular output and around the ascending aorta measure left ventricular output minus coronary flow (Rudolph and Heymann 1973). The fetal circulatory effects of drugs administered to the mother or fetus can be examined in these preparations. However, when drugs are administered to the mother, fetal responses may not be a direct effect, but may result from interference with uterine blood flow, causing fetal hypoxemia and possibly acidemia. Also, drugs that may depress the fetal circulation or constrict the umbilical-placental vessels could cause hypoxemia as a result of inadequate oxygen delivery. It is therefore advisable to examine the effects of drugs administered directly to the fetus as well as to the mother. Also, maternal cardiovascular variables such as blood pressure and heart rate, and particularly uterine blood flow, should be measured to assess maternal responses.

The radionuclide-labeled microsphere technique has greatly advanced the opportunity to examine fetal cardiovascular responses to drugs (Rudolph and Heymann 1967). Injection of microspheres with two different labels into an upper and lower limb vein with simultaneous sampling from upper and lower limb arteries allows measurement of cardiac output and blood flow to every organ and tissue and to the placenta. Currently, we can discriminate nine different gamma emitters, so that it is possible to obtain a control measurement and the effects of a drug at three different concentrations, if desired. The changes in vascular resistance in each organ can be assessed.

Some of the effects of drugs on the central nervous system can be examined by implanting leads to measure electrocortical activity or electroocular activity and limb or nuchal muscle movement (Ruckebusch et al. 1976).

The effects of drugs on renal function can readily be examined in the preparation we reported (Iwamoto and Rudolph 1983). Renal blood flow and urinary output, as well as urinary electrolyte composition, can be examined. Biochemical and endocrine effects of drugs can be studied by measuring plasma concentrations of metabolic substrates or hormones.

This review indicates that there have been considerable advances in the ability to study pharmacokinetics and pharmacodynamics of drugs in the fetus and mother during pregnancy. At present, the pregnant sheep preparation provides a useful model for drug studies. It must be appreciated, however, that there are important species differences in placental function. Furthermore, the state of maturation of the developing fetus varies greatly in different species at the time of birth. It is therefore not appropriate to assume that drug effects can be compared at similar proportions of the total gestational period.

REFERENCES

Berman, W., Jr.; Goodlin, R.C.; Heymann, M.A.; and Rudolph, A.M. The measurement of umbilical blood flow in fetal lambs in utero. J Appl Physiol 39:1056-1059, 1975.

Bristow, J.; Rudolph, A.M.; and Itskovitz, J. A preparation for studying liver blood flow, oxygen consumption, and metabolism in the fetal lamb in utero. J Dev Physiol 3:255-266, 1981.

Cosmi, E.V. Drugs, anesthetics and the fetus. In: Scarpelli, E.M., ed. Reviews in Perinatal Medicine. Vol. I. Baltimore: University Park Press, 1976. pp. 191-253.

Dutton, G.J. Developmental aspects of drug conjugations with special reference to glucuronidation. Am Rev Pharmacol Toxicol 18:17, 1978.

Edelstone, D.I., and Rudolph, A.M. Preferential streaming of ductus venosus blood to the brain and heart in fetal lambs. Am J Physiol 237:H724-H729, 1979.

Edelstone, D.I.; Rudolph, A.M.; and Heymann, M.A. Liver and ductus venosus blood flows in fetal lambs in utero. Circ Res 42:426-433, 1978.

Faber, J.J. Diffusional exchange between foetus and mother as a function of the physical properties of the diffusing materials. In: Proceedings of the Sir Joseph Barcroft Centenary Symposium: Foetal and Neonatal Physiology. Cambridge: Cambridge University Press, 1973. pp. 306-327.

Fouron, J.C. Dynamics of the placental transfer of digoxin in the dog. Biol Neonate 23:116-122, 1973.

Heymann, M.A.; Payne, B.D.; Hoffman, J.I.E.; and Rudolph, A.M. Blood flow measurements with radionuclide-labeled particles. Prog Cardiovasc Dis 20:55-79, 1977.

Iwamoto, H.S., and Rudolph, A.M. Chronic renal venous catheterization in fetal sheep. Am J Physiol 245:H524-H527, 1983.

Mellor, D.J. Investigations of fluid spaces of the sheep conceptus. In: Nathanielsz, P.W., ed. Animal Models in Fetal Medicine. Vol. I. Amsterdam: Elsevier/North-Holland Biomedical Press, 1980. pp. 59-106.

Meschia, G.; Cotter, J.R.; Makowski, E.L.; and Barron, D. Simultaneous measurement of uterine and umbilical blood flows and oxygen uptakes. Q J Exp Physiol 52:1-18, 1966.

Mirkin, B.L. Drug distribution in pregnancy. In: Boreus, L.O., ed. Fetal Pharmacology. New York: Raven Press, 1973. pp. 1-28.

Morishima, H.O.; Heymann, M.A.; Rudolph, A.M.; and Barrett, C.T. Toxicity of lidocaine in the fetal and newborn lamb and its relationship to asphyxia. Am J Obstet Gynecol 112:72-79, 1972.

Morishima, H.O.; Heymann, M.A.; Rudolph, A.M.; Barrett, C.T.; and James, L.S. Transfer of lidocaine across the sheep placenta to the fetus. Am J Obstet Gynecol 122:581-588, 1975.

Moya, F., and Thorndike, V. Passage of drugs across the placenta. Am J Obstet Gynecol 84:1778-1797, 1962.

Oakes, G.K.; Walker, A.M.; Ehrenkranz, R.A.; Cafalo, R.C.; and Chez, R.A. Uteroplacental blood flow during hyperthermia with and without respiratory alkalosis. J Appl Physiol 41:197-201, 1976.

Reuss, M.L., and Rudolph, A.M. Distribution and recirculation of umbilical and systemic venous blood flow in fetal lambs during hypoxia. J Dev Physiol 2:71-84, 1980.

Ruckebusch, Y.; Graujoux, M.; and Eghbali, B. Placental transfer of central nervous system depressants in sheep. Eur J Pharmacol 37:193-196, 1976.

Rudolph, A. M. Hepatic and ductus venosus blood flows during fetal life. Hepatology 3:254-258, 1983.

Rudolph, A.M., and Heymann, M.A. The circulation of the fetus in utero. Circ Res 21:163-184, 1967.

Rudolph, A.M., and Heymann, M.A. Control of the foetal circulation. In: Proceedings of the Sir Joseph Barcroft Centenary Symposium: Foetal and Neonatal Physiology. Cambridge: Cambridge University Press, 1973. pp. 89-111.

Rudolph, A.M., and Heymann, M.A. Methods for studying the circulation of the fetus in utero. In: Nathanielsz, P.W., ed. Animal Models in Fetal Medicine. Vol. I. Amsterdam: Elsevier/North-Holland Biomedical Press, 1980. pp. 1-57.

Schifferli, P.Y., and Caldeyro-Barcia, R. Effects of atropine and beta-adrenergic drugs on the heart rate of the human fetus. In: Boreus, L.O., ed. Fetal Pharmacology. New York: Raven Press, 1973. pp. 259-279.

Schneider, H.; Panigel, M.; and Dancis, J. Transfer across the perfused human placenta of antipyrine, sodium and leucine. Am J Obstet Gynecol 114:822-828, 1972.

Szeto, H.H.; Mann, L.I.; Bhaktharathsalan, A.; Liu, M.; and Inturrisi, C.E. Meperidine pharmacokinetics in the maternal-fetal unit. J Pharmacol Exp Ther 206:448-459, 1978.

Warkany, J., and Takacs, E. Experimental production of congenital malformations in rats by salicylate poisoning. Am J Pathol 35:315-331, 1959.

Young, W.P.; Creasy, R.K.; and Rudolph, A.M. Catheterization of the common umbilical vein for chronic fetal lamb studies. J Appl Physiol 37:620-621, 1974.

AUTHOR

Abraham M. Rudolph, M.D.
Professor of Pediatrics, Physiology, and
Obstetrics, Gynecology, and Reproductive Sciences
Neider Professor of Pediatric Cardiology
School of Medicine
University of California
San Francisco, California 94143

Biotransformations of Drugs and Foreign Chemicals in the Human Fetal-Placental Unit

M.R. Juchau

Prenatal drug biotransformation has attracted investigative attention since the late 1950s (Fouts and Adamson 1959; Jondorf et al. 1959) when it was recognized that differences between mature and developing organisms, in terms of their responses to the pharmacologic/toxicologic actions of drugs, could be due (at least in part) to developmental differences in biotransformation. The common biotransformation pathways for drugs and foreign chemicals are presented in table 1. Early studies on fetal drug metabolism primarily focused on hepatic tissues because the liver was recognized as the principal site of drug biotransformation reactions in adult animals. When compared in vitro with hepatic tissues from mature experimental animals, the corresponding tissues from fetuses and neonates exhibited extremely low or, in many cases, undetectable drug biotransforming activities. Based primarily on studies in rats, mice, rabbits, and guinea pigs, the concept arose that the drug biotransforming capacity of prenatal animals was virtually negligible. Early studies of fetal and neonatal drug biotransformation were reviewed by Brodie and Maickel (1962) and Fouts and Hart (1965). This concept (absence of prenatal drug biotransformation) persisted until the early 1970s when it was discovered independently, in three separate laboratories (Pelkonen et al. 1971a, 1971b; Rane and Ackerman 1972; Rane and Sjöqvist 1972; Juchau 1971; Juchau et al. 1972; Juchau and Pedersen 1973), that the human fetal liver and adrenal gland contained enzymes capable of catalyzing various monooxygenation reactions--reactions for one of the common biotransformation pathways of drugs and foreign chemicals (table 1), at reasonable respectable rates and at fairly early stages of gestation. Several reviews of these findings also have appeared in the literature (Pelkonen 1973, 1979, 1980a, 1980b, 1982; Yaffe and Juchau 1974; Rane et al. 1973; Juchau et al. 1980; Juchau 1980a).

Almost simultaneously, it was discovered that human placental tissues exhibited the capacity to biotransform drugs via each of the major metabolic pathways. Possibly the most striking aspect of placental drug biotransformation was the remarkably increased monooxygenase activities observed in placentas of tobacco smokers. Such increases were observed primarily in placentas delivered near term and contrasted with a relative

TABLE 1. Common biotransformation pathways and enzymes involved in biotransformation

PATHWAY	ENZYMES
I. Oxidation	I. Oxidoreductases
a) Monooxygenation	a1) Cytochrome P-450-dependent systems
	a2) Flavin-dependent monooxygenases
b) Dioxygenation	b) Dioxygenases
c) Dehydrogenation	c) Dehydrogenases
d) Peroxidation	d) Peroxidases
e) Monoamine oxidation	e) Monoamine oxidases
II. Reduction	II. Oxidoreductases
a) Nitro groups	a) Nitro reductases
b) Azo linkages	b) Azo reductases
c) Epoxides	c) Epoxide reductases
d) Carbonyl groups	d) Dehydrogenases
e) Unsaturated carbon-carbon bonds	e) Dehydrogenases
III. Hydrolysis	III. Hydrolases
a) Carboxylic acid esters	a) Esterases
b) Amides/peptides	b) Amidases
c) Sulphate esters	c) Sulphatases
d) Glucuronic acid esters	d) Glucuronidases
e) Epoxides	e) Epoxide hydrolases
IV. Conjugation	IV. Transferases
a) Glycosylation	a) Glycosyl transferases
1. Glucuronidation	1. Glucuronosyl transferases
2. Riboside formation	2. Ribosyl transferases
3. Glucoside formation	3. Glucosyl transferases
b) Sulphation	b) Sulphokinases
c) Acylation	c) Acyl transferases
1. Acetylation	1. Acetyl transferases
2. Glycine/glutamine conjugation	2. Amino acid transferases
d) Glutathione conjugation	d) Glutathione transferases
e) Methylation	e) Methyl transferases

lack of response during the first third of gestation. Fetal livers and adrenal glands also appeared not to respond significantly to inducing agents present in tobacco smoke between weeks 7 to 20 of gestation. Aspects of these research findings have been reviewed on numerous occasions. (For recent reviews, see Juchau 1980b, 1982, 1984; Chao and Juchau 1983; Juchau and Rettie, in press).

PHARMACOLOGIC SIGNIFICANCE

A somewhat disturbing aspect of the finding of comparatively high monooxygenase activities in human placental and fetal tissues is the indication provided by somewhat preliminary research that various enzymes deemed extremely important for bioinactivation of drugs and chemicals are present in low to negligible levels in each of the three aforementioned tissues (but particularly the placenta). They also appear to remain at low levels following exposure to inducing agents. Of principal concern is the low to negligible complement of glucuronyl transferases (in all fetal and placental tissues), enzymes which play a prime role in terminating the biologic effects of drugs and other chemicals. Activities of other conjugating enzymes may also be low, although no generalizations should be made at this time because of the fact that relatively high activities can be observed depending upon the substrate under investigation, the tissue preparation being studied, the stage of gestation, exposure to inducing agents, and a multitude of other genetic, physiological, and environmental factors known to affect rates of conjugation.

Under conditions in which the tissue monooxygenase activities are comparatively high, it can be shown that enzymes from each of these three organs will catalyze the conversion of promutagens to mutagenic intermediary metabolites (Jones et al. 1977; Juchau et al. 1978, 1980; Juchau 1980a). Other bioactivation reactions also have been documented (Rollins et al. 1979; Pelkonen 1979, 1982). The toxicologic significance of these observations is not fully understood at present but would suggest that after exposure of pregnant women to drugs or chemicals, steady-state levels of reactive, toxic intermediates would tend to be high in fetal and placental tissues with high ratios of monooxygenase to conjugating activities. Considerable research must be performed in order to understand the implications of regulatory increases in xenobiotic monooxygenation in the fetal-placental unit. From the viewpoint of toxicologic effects of drugs and chemicals, the influence of such changes will undoubtedly vary depending on the toxic chemical under consideration. It is important to emphasize that we are now in possession of only the barest framework of knowledge of xenobiotic biotransformation in human fetal and placental tissues and that it is entirely premature to make predictions concerning the metabolic fate of a given chemical within the human fetal-placental unit based on currently available information. Recently, we discovered (Juchau et al. 1982; Namkung et al. 1983a, 1983b; Omiecinski et al. 1980) that additions of micromolar quantities of hematin to reaction mixtures containing fetal or placental tissues as enzyme source would increase rates of monooxygenation by as much or more than a hundredfold, depending upon reaction conditions and the tissue under investigation. The mechanism for elicitation of these remarkable increases has not yet been elucidated, but evidence accumulated to date suggests that the phenomenon may reflect a highly important, short-term mode of regulation of P-450-dependent monooxygenation reactions. In view of the implications for generation of toxic reactive intermediates, it would seem important to gain a much firmer understanding of the phenomenon. We are currently pursuing studies of "hematin-mediated" regulation of P-450-dependent monooxygenase activities in fetal and placental tissues with the following working hypothesis:

> Extrahepatic tissues of mature animals and both hepatic and extrahepatic tissues of immature (prenatal and neonatal) animals (including human and nonhuman primates) contain significant pools of apocytochrome P-450 isozymes which, under normal circumstances, exhibit a relatively low affinity for the corresponding hematin prosthetic group. Following contact with certain small organic chemicals (not necessarily xenobiotics, as hydroxylation of estradiol 17ß also appears subject to this regulatory mode), interaction of the apocytochrome with the chemical and/or its metabolite(s) results in a conformational change in the apocytochrome(s) which increases the affinity for its hematin prosthetic group. The increased affinity, in turn, results in an increased steady-state level of active holocytochrome(s) and thus, a marked increase in the corresponding P-450-dependent monooxygenase activities.

Although the hypothesis remains unproven, we have provided substantial evidence to rule out a large number of possible alternative hypotheses and also have found that all data obtained to date are consistent with the stated hypothesis. In addition, we have been able to show (Giachelli et al. 1984) that embryonic tissues contain unusually high quantities of mRNA which serve as template for P-450 synthesis, suggesting the possibility that correspondingly high levels of inactive apocytochrome may also be present prenatally. In view of the importance of the role of P-450-dependent monooxygenation in the generation of reactive intermediates and in the potential serious toxic effects of such intermediates, it is felt that pursuit of these questions could provide considerable light on mechanisms of chemically initiated toxicity in the fetal-placental unit.

It should be emphasized, however, that our current understanding of drug biotransformation in the human fetal-placental unit is very primitive. It is not possible to predict the metabolic fate of drugs and foreign chemicals within that unit--even for chemicals that have received some investigative attention. For obvious reasons, investigators have utilized model substrates (primarily) for the study of the metabolic capabilities of the pertinent human fetal and placental tissues. Thus, specific information on most drugs of abuse is not available at present, nor is it possible to predict their biotransformational fate within the fetal-placental unit. Understandably, in view of the ethical questions involved, progress in the area has been rather slow, with only a few published articles appearing each year. For these and other reasons, our understanding of the effects of drugs of abuse on the prenatal organism (particularly in terms of the more subtle, nonmorphologic and/or long-term effects) is incomplete at best. Future research, however, will undoubtedly help to clarify many of the currently existing questions.

SUMMARY

Several communications pertaining to research on human fetal drug biotransformation have appeared in the literature in the past 3 to 4 years (Aranda et al. 1979; Cresteil et al. 1982; Pacifici et al. 1981; Pacifici and Rane 1982, 1983; Schroeter and Amon 1983). In general, research in this area has produced no major recent surprises, but it has confirmed, extended, and supported the earliest findings through those of the mid-1970s and has served to expand our understanding of these important systems. The important aspects of our current knowledge may be summarized very briefly as follows:

1. Each of the major drug metabolic reactions (oxidations, reductions, hydrolyses, and conjugations) can be catalyzed at generally low rates by enzymes present in human fetal and placental tissues.

2. Reaction rates appear, in general, to increase with advancing gestational age.

3. Placental xenobiotic-biotransforming monooxygenases display a high sensitivity to the effects of MC-type (methylcholanthrene) but not PB-type (phenobarbital) inducing agents during the later stages of gestation. Responsivity is minimal during early gestation.

4. Monooxygenases in other fetal tissues (liver, adrenal gland, etc.) appear to respond minimally to inducing agents, at least during the earlier stages of gestation.

5. Glucuronyl transferase activities appear to be very low in all fetal and placental tissues.

6. Epoxide hydrolase, glutathione S-transferase, and sulfotransferase (and perhaps others) activities can be relatively high in prenatal primate hepatic tissues but, at present, are difficult to predict. Some of these may respond to environmental inducers <u>in situ</u>, but solid evidence for this is still lacking.

7. Monooxygenases in all fetal and placental tissues (with the exception of the liver in certain species) appear subject to a hematin-mediated regulation of activity. Extremely large increases have been observed.

8. Enzymes/enzyme systems present in human fetal and placental tissues can catalyze the generation of reactive intermediary metabolites capable of covalently binding to biomacromolecules and inducing bacterial mutations.

9. In terms of substrates attacked by human tissue monooxygenases, the fetal hepatic enzyme exhibits a rather broad specificity, the fetal adrenal gland exhibits a narrower specificity, and the human placenta exhibits an even narrower specificity.

10. In comparison with hepatic systems from adult male rodents, human fetal and placental tissues are virtually unexplored with respect to knowledge of drug biotransformation.

REFERENCES

Aranda, J.V.; Louridas, A.T.; Vitullo, B.B.; Aldridge, P.T.A.; and Haber, R. Metabolism of theophylline to caffeine in human fetal liver. Science 206:1319-1321, 1979.

Brodie, B.B., and Maickel, R.P. Comparative biochemistry of drug metabolism. In: Brodie, B.B., and Erdos, E.G., eds. Proceedings of the First International Pharmacological Meeting. Vol. 6. Metabolic Factors Controlling the Duration of Drug Action. Oxford: Pergamon Press, 1962. pp. 229-324.

Chao, S.T., and Juchau, M.R. Placental drug metabolism. In: Johnson, E.M., and Kochhar, D.M., eds. Teratogenesis and Reproductive Toxicology (Handbook of Experimental Pharmacology). Vol. 65. New York: Springer Verlag, 1983. pp. 31-49.

Cresteil, T.; Beaune, P.; Kremers, P.; Flinois, J.; and Leroux, J. Drug metabolizing enzymes in human fetal liver: Partial resolution of multiple cytochromes P-450. Pediatr Pharmacol 2:199-207, 1982.

Fouts, J.R., and Adamson, R.H. Drug metabolism in the newborn rabbit. Science 129:807-898, 1959.

Fouts, J.R., and Hart, L.G. Hepatic drug metabolism during the perinatal period. Ann NY Acad Sci 123:245-251, 1965.

Giachelli, C.M.; Juchau, M.R.; and Omiecinski, C.J. Expression of cytochrome P-450 and epoxide hydrolase messenger RNA in developing rat embryos. Fed Proc 43:122, 1984.

Jondorf, W.R.; Maickel, R.P.; and Brodie, B.B. Inability of newborn mice and guinea pigs to metabolize drugs. Biochem Pharmacol 1:352-354, 1959.

Jones, A.H.; Fantel, A.G.; Kocan, R.A.; and Juchau, M.R. Bioactivation of procarcinogens to mutagens in human fetal and placental tissues. Life Sci 21:1831-1836, 1977.

Juchau, M.R. Drug biotransformation in the human fetus: Nitro group reduction. Arch Int Pharmacodyn Ther 194:346-358, 1971.

Juchau, M.R. Enzymatic bioactivation and inactivation of chemical teratogens and transplacental carcinogens and mutagens. In: Juchau, M.R., ed. The Biochemical Basis of Chemical Teratogenesis. New York: Elsevier Press, 1980a. pp.63-95.

Juchau, M.R. Drug biotransformation in the placenta. Pharmacol Ther 8:501-524, 1980b.

Juchau, M.R. The role of the placenta in developmental toxicology. In: Snell, K., ed. Developmental Toxicology. London: Croom-Helm, 1982. pp. 189-209.

Juchau, M.R. Placental drug metabolism with respect to transplacental carcinogenesis. In: Reznik-Schuller, H.M., ed. Comparative Perinatal Carcinogenesis. New York: CRC Press, 1984. pp. 117-137.

Juchau, M.R., and Pedersen, M.G. Drug biotransformation reactions in the human fetal adrenal gland. Life Sci 12:193-204, 1973.

Juchau, M.R., and Rettie, A.E. The metabolic role of the placenta. In: Fabro, S.E., and Scialli, A.R., eds. Principles of Drug and Chemical Action in Pregnancy. New York: Marcel-Dekker Inc., in press.

Juchau, M.R.; Pedersen, M.G.; and Symms, K.G. Hydroxylation of 3,4-benzpyrene in human fetal tissue homogenates. Biochem Pharmacol 21:2269-2272, 1972.

Juchau, M.R.; Jones, A.H.; Namkung, M.J.; and DiGiovanni, J. Extrahepatic bioactivation of 7,12-dimethylbenz(α)anthracene and benzo(α)pyrene man fetal tissues. In: Jones, P.W., and Freudenthal, R.I., eds. Carcinogenesis Vol. III: Polynuclear Aromatic Hydrocarbons. New York: Raven Press, 1978. pp. 361-370.

Juchau, M.R.; Chao, S.T.; and Omiecinski, C.J. Drug metabolism by the human fetus. Clin Pharmacokinet 5:320-339, 1980.

Juchau, M.R.; Omiecinski, C.J.; and Namkung, M.J. Hematin-mediated increases in P-450-dependent monooxygenation reactions: An apparent short-term regulatory mechanism. In: Sato, R., and Kato, R., eds. Microsomes, Drug Oxidations and Drug Toxicities. New York: Wiley-Interscience, 1982. pp. 371-381.

Namkung, M.J.; Chao, S.T.; and Juchau, M.R. Placental monooxygenation: characteristics and partial purification of a hematin-activated human placental monooxygenase. Drug Metab Dispos 11:10-15, 1983a.

Namkung, M.J.; Faustman-Watts, E.M.; and Juchau, M.R. Hematin-mediated increases in benzo(α)pyrene monooxygenation in maternal, fetal and placental tissues of inducible and non-inducible mouse strains. Dev Pharmacol Ther 6:199-207, 1983b.

Omiecinski, C.J.; Chao, S.T.; and Juchau, M.R. Modulation of monooxygenases activity by hematin and 7,8-benzoflavone in fetal tissues of rats, rabbits and humans. Dev Pharmacol Ther 1:90-100, 1980.

Pacifici, G.M., and Rane, A. Renal glucuronidation of morphine in the human fetus. Acta Pharmacol Toxicol 50:155-160, 1982.

Pacifici, G.M., and Rane, A. Epoxide hydrolase in human fetal liver. Pharmacol 26:241-248, 1983.

Pacifici, G.M.; Norlin, A.; and Rane, A. Glutathione S-transferase in human fetal liver. Biochem Pharmacol 30:3367-3371, 1981 .

Pelkonen, O. Drug metabolism in human fetal tissues. Life Sci 13:1163-1180, 1973.

Pelkonen, O. Prenatal and neonatal development of drug and carcinogen metabolism. In: Estabrook, R., and Lindelaub, J., eds. The Induction of Drug Metabolism. Stuttgart: F.K. Schattauer Verlag, 1979. pp. 507-516.

Pelkonen, O. Environmental influences on human fetal and placental xenobiotic metabolism. Eur J Clin Pharmacol 18:17-24, 1980a.

Pelkonen, O. Biotransformation of xenobiotics in the fetus. Pharmacol Ther 10:261-281, 1980b.

Pelkonen, O. The differentiation of drug metabolism in relation to developmental toxicity. In: Snell, K., ed. Developmental Toxicology. London: Croom-Helm, 1982. pp. 167-188.

Pelkonen, O.; Vorne, M.; Jouppila, P.; and Karki, N.T. Metabolism of chlorpromazine and p-nitrobenzoic acid in the liver, intestine and kidney of the human fetus. Acta Pharmacol Toxicol 29:284-294, 1971a.

Pelkonen, O.; Arvela, P.; and Karki, N.T. 3,4-Benzpyrene and N-methylaniline metabolizing enzymes in immature human fetus and placenta. Acta Pharmacol Toxicol 30:385-395, 1971b.

Rane, A., and Ackerman, E. Metabolism of ethylmorphine and aniline in human fetal liver. Clin Pharmacol Ther 13:663-670, 1972.

Rane, A., and Sjöqvist, F. Drug metabolism in the human fetus and newborn infant. Pediatr Clin North Am 19:37-49, 1972.

Rane, A.; Sjöqvist, F.; and Orrenius, S. Drugs and fetal metabolism. Clin Pharmacol Ther 14:666-672, 1973.
Rollins, D.E.; Von Bahr, C.; Glaumann, H.; Moldeus, P.; and Rane, A. Acetaminophen: Potentially toxic metabolite formed by human fetal and adult liver microsomes and isolated fetal liver cells. Science 205:1414-1416, 1979.
Schroeter, A., and Amon, I. Acetylsalicylic acid esterase activity in human fetal organs during development. Int J Biol Res Preg 1:31-34, 1983.
Yaffe, S.J., and Juchau, M.R. Perinatal pharmacology. Annu Rev Pharmacol Toxicol 14:219-238, 1974.

AUTHOR

M.R. Juchau, Ph.D.
Department of Pharmacology
University of Washington SJ-30
Seattle, WA 98195

Pharmacokinetics of Drugs and Metabolites in the Maternal-Placental-Fetal Unit: General Principles

Laurene H. Wang, Abraham M. Rudolph, and Leslie Z. Benet

Drug use during pregnancy may result in both pharmacologic and toxicologic drug effects in the fetus. Prenatal pharmacology defines the therapeutic use of drugs to treat fetal diseases in utero; while prenatal toxicology evaluates the risks of drug exposure to the developing fetus. To correctly assess the pharmacologic and toxicologic effects of a drug, one must examine both the pharmacodynamics and pharmacokinetics of the drug and its metabolites. Pharmacodynamic parameters which specify the interaction of a drug or its metabolites with certain specific receptors and the elucidation of their modes of action determine whether the drug or its metabolites possess pharmacological or toxicological potential in the fetus. On the other hand, pharmacokinetic parameters which characterize the disposition of the drug and its metabolites in the maternal-placental-fetal unit are of utmost importance in determining whether an active form of the drug can reach the fetus, after maternal administration, at a sufficient concentration and for an adequate period to induce pharmacological or toxicological effects during the prenatal period. Therefore, pharmacokinetic studies in the maternal-placental-fetal unit which evaluate the rate and extent of drug exposure to the fetus play an important role in developmental pharmacology and toxicology.

An index of relative exposure of the fetus to the drug taken by the mother has been defined as the ratio of the total area under the drug concentration versus time curve for the fetus to that for the mother after a single-dose administration (Levy and Hayton 1973). If multiple doses of a drug are administered, the index of relative exposure of the fetus to the drug can be determined by the ratio of the steady-state drug concentration in the fetus to that in the mother. Since the metabolite of a drug is, in many cases, the active species responsible for a pharmacologic or toxicologic effect, the concentrations of the metabolite should then be measured to determine the fetal metabolite exposure. In addition, plasma protein binding measurements should also be determined because the unbound drug is generally believed to be the moiety that elicits a pharmacologic or toxicologic action. The factors affecting the rate, extent, and duration of exposure of a drug or its metabolites to the fetus include the absorption, distribution, and elimination of the drug in the mother; the distribution and elimination of the drug metabolites in the mother; the transfer of the drug and its metabolites across the placenta;

the metabolism of the drug or its metabolites in the placenta; and the distribution and elimination of the drug and its metabolites in the fetus. Theoretical considerations of all the above processes of drug disposition in the maternal-placental-fetal unit are presented in this chapter. Pharmacokinetic experiments which have been utilized to assess appropriate pharmacokinetic parameters for characterizing the kinetic processes are also discussed.

PHARMACOKINETIC STUDIES DURING PREGNANCY

Pharmacokinetic studies in humans during pregnancy are usually limited to a single point determination of drug concentrations in the mother and the fetus (umbilical cord blood) immediately following delivery. These determinations are carried out in different subjects, at different times after drug administration, and usually under different conditions. Consequently, pharmacokinetic characterization of drug disposition in the maternal-placental-fetal unit derived from these studies is extremely difficult and by no means is definitive in reflecting in utero condition. Based on theoretical considerations, computer simultations using various pharmacokinetic models have been undertaken to predict the time course of drug concentrations in the mother and fetus (Levy and Hayton 1973; Gillette 1977). Nonetheless, the most useful information can only be obtained from properly conducted experiments in which the time course of maternal plasma concentrations of drug and metabolites is followed after drug administration; and maternal, cord arterial, and venous blood samples and amniotic fluid are collected at the time of delivery (Rajchgot and MacLeod 1983). In addition, the plasma protein binding of the drug and its metabolites should also be determined.

Since drug studies in pregnant woman are ethically and medically prohibited, most multiple sample pharmacokinetic investigations of drugs and metabolites have been carried out in animals. Rats, mice, and rabbits have been frequently utilized with a single time sample obtained in both the mother and fetus at sacrifice. Pharmacokinetic analyses are then undertaken with combined data from many animals sacrificed at different times after dosing. A few multiple time sample studies have been carried out in monkeys, but the pregnant sheep has evolved as the most frequently used animal model.

The establishment of a chronically catheterized pregnant sheep model has allowed complete pharmacokinetic studies in the maternal-placental-fetal unit in utero. Surgical procedures are used to implant chronic indwelling catheters, enabling repeated sampling from various maternal and fetal blood vessels, from maternal and fetal bladders, and from amniotic and allantoic fluid cavities at predetermined time intervals after drug administration. Chronic studies with multiple dosing of a drug to the mother and kinetic studies with direct introduction of the drugs into the fetal circulation can also be readily carried out. Additionally, the pregnant ewe preparation permits pharmacokinetic studies on the developmental aspects of drug disposition in the maternal-placental-fetal unit. Therefore, the following discussion of the experimental methods utilized in prenatal pharmacokinetic studies will concentrate on the use of pregnant sheep as the animal model. However, comparative studies using different animal models are essential to gain a full understanding of the overall scheme of drug disposition in the maternal-placental-fetal unit.

Pharmacokinetic Models

Various compartmental models have been suggested for characterizing the kinetics of drug disposition in the maternal-placental-fetal unit during pregnancy (Levy and Hayton 1973; Krauer and Krauer 1977; Szeto 1982; Szeto et al. 1982; Rajchgot and MacLeod 1983; Gabrielsson and Paalzow 1983). To obtain the pharmacokinetic parameters which best describe the rate, extent, and duration of drug exposure to the fetus, all accountable kinetic processes must be considered when constructing the pharmacokinetic model. The compartmental model can be as complicated as that shown in figure 1 in which all possible physiological conditions of the system are considered. However, the practicality of a kinetic model is usually limited by the availability of sampling sites, and, thus the experimental data. Therefore, preliminary in vivo and in vitro experiments should always be performed to provide the basis for a particular model. Furthermore, model independent or noncompartmental methods should be utilized to substantiate the validity of the derived compartmental parameters using the proposed model. If the experimental results of both methods are not consistent, a model describing more complicated processes should then be proposed and tested.

At present, it appears that the simplest kinetic model would be a two-compartment (maternal and fetal) model with transplacental transfer and nontransplacental elimination occurring in both compartments (Szeto 1982). As depicted in figure 1, complicated situations arise when the drug is metabolized in the placenta, which constitutes a third compartment, or when the drug is transferred via nonplacental routes between the fetus and the mother. This is exemplified by the reversible diffusion of the drug between the amniotic fluid and the mother across the chorioallantoic membranes (Mellor 1980), the reversible diffusion of the drug between the amniotic fluid and the fetus across the fetal skin, chorioamnion, or respiratory epithelium (Seeds 1981; Carson et al. 1979; Dawes 1973), or the oral-renal-amniotic fluid recycling (Amon and Amon 1976). The pharmacokinetic scheme is further complicated when metabolite kinetics is considered. Overall, the significance of each process in a kinetic model depends upon its contribution to the overall estimation of the pharmacokinetic parameters which govern the rate, extent, and duration of drug exposure to the fetus.

Experimental Methods

Once a compartmental model is proposed for the disposition of a drug in the maternal-placental-fetal unit, the rate equations describing the change of drug concentration in each compartment can be written. When steady-state infusions of the drug into each compartment are carried out on separate occasions, the rate of change of drug concentration at steady state in each compartment is equal to zero for every infusion experiment. The drug concentration in each compartment at steady state and the infusion rate for each experiment allow one to determine the clearance of the drug for each process describing the disposition of the drug in the maternal-placental-fetal unit. A two-compartment open model with elimination from both the maternal and fetal compartments has been utilized by Szeto (1982) and Szeto et al. (1982) to determine the transplacental clearances from both sides of the placental membranes and the nontransplacental clearance from the mother and the fetus, as expressed in the following equations:

483-942 0 - 85 - 2 : QL 3

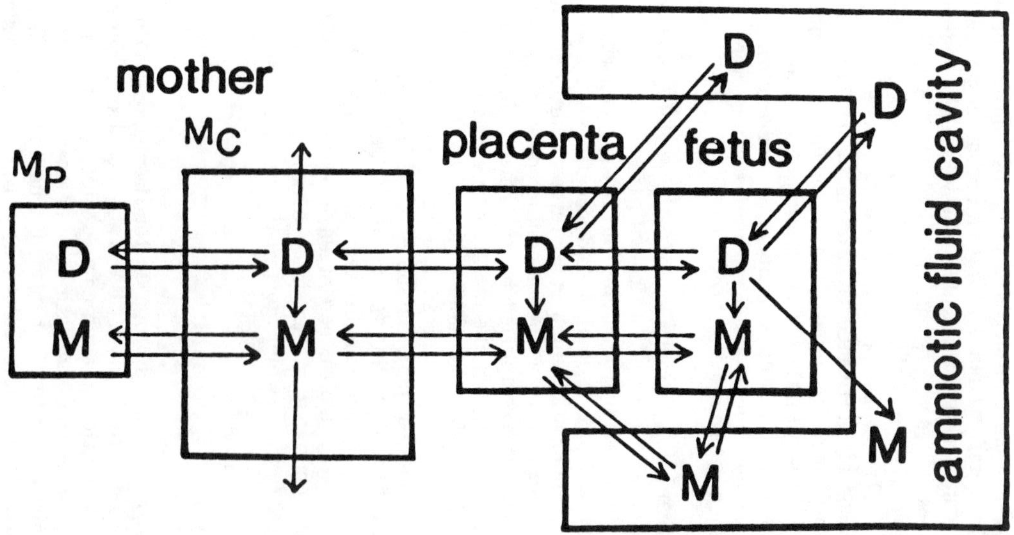

FIGURE 1. Schematic Representation of the Drug Transfer and Elimination Processes in the Mother, Placenta, and Fetus. M_C = maternal central compartment; M_P = maternal peripheral compartment; D = drug; and M = metabolite.

$$CL_{MF} = \frac{J'}{\left(\frac{C_M \cdot C_F'}{C_F} - C_M'\right)} \quad (1)$$

$$CL_{FM} = \frac{J}{\left(\frac{C_F' \cdot C_M}{C_M'} - C_F\right)} \quad (2)$$

$$CL_{Mo} = \frac{CL_{FM} \cdot C_F'}{C_M'} - CL_{MF} \quad (3)$$

$$CL_{Fo} = \frac{CL_{MF} \cdot C_M}{C_F} - CL_{FM} \quad (4)$$

Where CL_{MF} and CL_{FM} are the respective transplacental clearances of drug from the mother to the fetus and from the fetus to the mother; CL_{Mo} and CL_{Fo} are the respective nontransplacental elimination clearances of drug from the mother and the fetus; J and J' are the respective infusion rates of the drug into the maternal and the fetal compartments; C_M and C_F are the respective steady-state drug concentrations in the mother and the fetus after maternal infusion; and C_M' and C_F' are the respective steady-state drug concentrations in the mother and the fetus after the fetal infusion.

When experimental techniques permit, direct measurement of these clearance terms should be undertaken independently in the mother, placenta, and fetus to verify the credibility of the clearance terms obtained with the compartmental model method. With catheterization of uterine and umbilical veins in addition to the maternal and fetal femoral arteries, it is possible to determine clearances across the placenta from either side using the extraction ratio method by measuring the arterial and venous drug concentrations across the placenta and the uterine and umbilical venous blood flow rates with radiolabeled microspheres (Rudolph and Heymann 1980). The placental clearance determined by the extraction ratio method consists of both the transfer clearance across the placenta and the metabolic clearance, if any, in the placenta; while the transplacental clearances (CL_{MF} and CL_{FM}) obtained from the two-compartment model method solely represent the transfer clearances. (For the two-compartment model method, placental metabolic clearance would be included in the CL_{Mo} and CL_{Fo} terms.) If placental metabolism does not exist, clearance values obtained from both methods should be equal. In addition to the <u>in vitro</u> placental incubation experiments, the extraction ratio method provides justification for incorporating placental metabolism in the pharmacokinetic model.

The validity of the nontransplacental clearances in the mother and the fetus, calculated from the compartmental model method at steady state, can be verified by determining the metabolic and renal clearances of the drug in the mother and the fetus following single-dose administration of drug or metabolite to both the mother and fetus. If the drug metabolite(s) is (are) not transferred across the placenta, metabolic clearance(s) of the drug can be determined using the general methods described by Benet (1984). Thus, the disposition of the drug metabolite(s) in the maternal-placental-fetal unit should be characterized prior to the assessment of metabolic clearances of the drug in the mother and the fetus. A valid nontransplacental clearance obtained from the model dependent method should be equal to the sum of the clearances of the drug via all elimination routes (metabolism and excretion) other than placental transfer.

Preliminary experiments to provide evidence of drug transfer through nonplacental routes can be performed by administering single bolus doses of the drug respectively into the mother, fetus, amniotic fluid cavity, and allantoic fluid cavity on separate occasions. Samples are collected from the amniotic fluid and allantoic fluid cavities, the maternal femoral artery and uterine vein, and the fetal femoral artery and umbilical vein. The rate and extent of drug appearance at each sampling site, e.g., the lag time, the peak time, peak concentration, and total area under the concentration-time curve, can then be compared between the sampling sites and between the studies. These comparisons allow one to better understand the mechanism of drug transfer via nonplacental routes, and they serve as a basis for upgrading a kinetic model to incorporate all the necessary transfer routes for describing drug disposition in the maternal-placental-fetal unit.

Metabolite Kinetics in the Fetus

Drug metabolism in the fetus has been extensively studied using in vitro enzyme preparations (Pelkonen 1980; Dutton and Leakey 1982). Very limited literature information is available regarding the in utero drug metabolism in the fetus. Since an understanding of the metabolic activation and deactivation pathways in the fetus is essential to determine drug effects and toxicity during the prenatal period (Lucier et al. 1979), studies of in utero drug metabolism in the fetus are indispensable in prenatal pharmacology and toxicology. Pharmacokinetics along with appropriate animal models provide us with a very useful tool to investigate fetal drug metabolism in utero.

A drug metabolite detected in the fetal circulation after drug administration to the mother may not reflect the ability of the fetus to metabolize the drug. Further investigation is required to determine whether the metabolite found in the fetus originates from fetal metabolic activity or results from transfer of the metabolite from the mother across the placenta. In addition, if a metabolite is formed in the fetus, the distribution and elimination processes of the metabolite in the fetus must be examined in order to quantitate the fetal metabolic activity in utero. To this end, a single dose of the metabolite can be administered to the mother to determine whether placental transfer of the metabolite occurs. The metabolite should then be given to the fetus to examine the fetal disposition of the metabolite. Upon the identification of all elimination processes of the metabolite in the maternal-placental-fetal unit, rate equations describing the change of the metabolite concentration in the fetus can be written. As stated earlier, if the metabolite is not transferable across the placenta, the formation clearance for the metabolite (or metabolic clearance of the drug) can be determined using general pharmacokinetic methods (Benet 1984). An example of these methods will be demonstrated in the following section of this paper. If the metabolite is formed in the fetus and is transferred across the placenta from both sides, computer simulations and data fitting may be helpful in obtaining the formation clearance for the metabolite in the fetus. Studies of in utero metabolite kinetics in the fetus at different gestational ages can then be carried out to investigate the prenatal development of various metabolic pathways.

EXAMPLE OF PHARMACOKINETIC STUDIES DURING PREGNANCY

We have chosen acetaminophen as a model compound to carry out pharmacokinetic studies of drug disposition in the sheep maternal-placental-fetal unit. These studies are presented here to illustrate the concepts and methods discussed above. The primary reasons for choosing acetaminophen are: (1) acetaminophen is the most widely administered nonprescription drug during pregnancy and clinicians frequently question the safety of its use in pregnant women; (2) acetaminophen is mostly glucuronidated and sulfated in various animal species and can thus serve as a model substrate to study the prenatal development of the two conjugation pathways; and (3) pure acetaminophen conjugates can be chemically synthesized in sufficient quantities for metabolite kinetic studies in the mother and the fetus.

Single bolus doses of acetaminophen were first administered intravenously (i.v.) into the mother and the fetus on two separate occasions (Wang et al. 1983). Acetaminophen was found to be transferred across the placenta from both sides of the membrane and its half-life was about 1 hour in both the mother and fetus. Both acetaminophen glucuronide and sulfate were measurable in the fetus and their concentrations gradually increased until the end of study. Both conjugates stayed in the fetal circulation for a much longer period than in the maternal circulation. Compared to acetaminophen glucuronide, acetaminophen sulfate had a higher concentration in the fetus but a lower concentration in the mother. This preliminary study revealed the bidirectional placental transfer of acetaminophen and the presence of its two conjugates in the fetus. Half-lives of acetaminophen and its conjugates in both the mother and the fetus were also determined. Acetaminophen glucuronide and sulfate were then administered i.v. simultaneously in single bolus doses into the mother and the fetus on separate occasions to examine the possibility of placental transfer of the two conjugates and to study the disposition of the two conjugates in the mother and the fetus (Wang et al. 1985a). Samples were collected from the maternal femoral artery and the uterine vein and bladder catheters; and from the fetal femoral artery and the umbilical vein and bladder catheters. It was found that acetaminophen glucuronide and sulfate were not transferred across the placenta from either side and that renal excretion is the predominant route of elimination for both conjugates in the mother and the fetus. Considering the glomerular filtration rate and the extent of plasma protein binding, we concluded that renal elimination of both conjugates was primarily through glomerular filtration in the fetus, but through renal tubular secretion in the mother. The increasing glomerular filtration rate with gestational age resulted in an increase of total (renal) clearances of both conjugates with gestational age. Steady-state volumes of distribution were determined for both conjugates in the fetus and were also found to be linearly related to the age of the fetus. This study demonstrated that the two conjugates detected in the fetal circulation following acetaminophen dosing originated from metabolic conjugation activities in the fetus, but not from placental transfer. Following the characterization of conjugates disposition in the fetus, it was then possible to quantitate conjugation activities in fetal lambs in utero using acetaminophen as the model substrate.

Since preliminary in vitro and in vivo data suggested negligible placental metabolism of acetaminophen, we proposed a two-compartment open model (Szeto 1982), with elimination from both the mother and fetus, to investigate the bidirectional placental transfer of acetaminophen and the total nontransplacental elimination of acetaminophen in the ewe and the fetal lamb (Wang et al. 1985b). Based on the data from steady-state i.v. infusions of acetaminophen into the mother and the fetus on separate occasions, the transplacental clearances from both sides of the membrane and the total nontransplacental clearances in the mother and the fetus were calculated using the equations stated above (1 to 4). The ratio of steady-state acetaminophen concentration, fetus to mother, after maternal infusion was found to be 0.77 and remained unchanged throughout the gestational age of the fetus. Transplacental clearances from mother to fetus and vice versa did not differ, indicating that acetaminophen is transferred across the placenta exclusively through passive diffusion since the plasma protein binding of acetaminophen is insignificant and comparable in both the mother and the fetus. The placental clearance was also determined using the extraction ratio method and found to approximate the transplacental clearances obtained from the compartmental model method, indicating that the model dependent method yields credible results for transplacental clearances, and that the placental metabolism is either nonexistent or negligible. The model independent total nontransplacental clearance of acetaminophen in the mother and the fetus were determined using the plasma and urine data. Since acetaminophen conjugates are not transferred across the placenta from either direction and renal excretion is the only elimination route for both conjugates (Wang et al. 1985a), the metabolic clearance of acetaminophen in the mother with respect to glucuronidation ($CL_{M,A \rightarrow G}$) or sulfation ($CL_{M,A \rightarrow S}$) was determined at steady state as the amount of the glucuronide or sulfate excreted in the urine divided by the area under the plasma acetaminophen concentration-time curve at steady state. The metabolic clearance in the fetus with regard to glucuronidation or sulfation was estimated based on the following equation:

$$CL_{F,A \rightarrow C} = \frac{V_{ssF,C} \cdot \int_{t_1}^{t_2} dC_{F,C} + \int_{t_1}^{t_2} dU_{F,C}}{\int_{t_1}^{t_2} C_{F,A} dt} \quad (5)$$

Where $CL_{F,A \to C}$ is the metabolic clearance of acetaminophen to a particular conjugate; $V_{ssF,C}$ is the steady-state volume of distribution of the conjugate in the fetus and is obtained from the previous conjugate dose experiments; $C_{F,C}$ and $C_{F,A}$ are the respective plasma conjugate and acetaminophen concentration in the fetus; and $U_{F,C}$ is the cumulative amount of the conjugate excreted in the fetal urine.

The sum of glucuronidation and sulfation clearances and the renal clearance of acetaminophen in the mother accounted for 98% of the nontransplacental clearance in the mother obtained from the compartmental model method. This provides further evidence of the validity of the two compartment model used for describing acetaminophen disposition in the sheep maternal-placental-fetal unit. Glucuronidation and sulfation activities in the fetus <u>in utero</u> were found to be 15% and 50% of the respective activities in the mother on a body weight basis. However, the sum of glucuronidation and sulfation clearances and renal clearance of acetaminophen cannot account for the overall nontransplacental clearance in the fetus obtained from the model dependent method. We speculate that diffusion of acetaminophen into the slow equilibrating amniotic fluid or metabolism of acetaminophen across the amnion, fetal intestine or lungs may partly explain this discrepancy. We now plan to collect both amniotic and allantoic fluids in addition to blood samples and to administer acetaminophen intra-amniotically and intra-allantoically to study the kinetics of acetaminophen disposition in the two fetal fluids and the possible drug transfer in relation to the maternal and fetal circulations. By these means, we hope to be able to propose a more sophisticated model to characterize the disposition of acetaminophen in the sheep maternal-placental-fetal unit.

FACTORS AFFECTING FETAL DRUG EXPOSURE

The factors which may influence the rate, extent, and duration of drug exposure to the fetus are essentially the factors that modify the pharmacokinetic parameters characterizing the absorption, distribution, metabolism, and elimination of the drug or/and its metabolites in the pregnant mother, the placenta, and the developing fetus. The determinants of fetal drug exposure during pregnancy are therefore categorized as the maternal, placental, and fetal factors. Several review articles on drug disposition in the maternal-placental-fetal unit have been published (Mirkin and Singh 1976; Krauer et al. 1980); Juchau and Faustman-Watts 1983; Bogaert and Thiery 1983), in which the maternal, placental, and fetal factors affecting fetal drug exposure have been discussed. Extensive and specific discussion of the maternal factors which modify the absorption, distribution, and elimination of the drug or/and its metabolites in pregnant women are presented in the articles by Krauer and Krauer (1977), Juchau and Faustman-Watts (1983), and Bogaert and Thiery (1983). Articles by Mirkin and Singh (1976), Juchau (1976), Nau and Liddiard (1978), and Goodman et al. (1982) specifically discuss placental metabolism of drugs and factors affecting placental transfer of drug or/and its metabolites. The distribution and elimination of drug or/and its metabolites in the fetus are specifically discussed in the articles by Mirkin and Singh (1976), Pelkonen (1980), Aranda and Stern (1983), Juchau and Faustman-Watts (1983), and Rajchgot and MacLeod (1983). Similar topics are addressed by Drs. Juchau and Miller in this volume. The following section summarizes the literature discussions and presents a brief review of the maternal, placental, and fetal factors affecting fetal drug exposure.

Maternal Factors

Absorption. The gastrointestinal absorption of drugs in pregnant women will be influenced by pregnancy-related physiological changes, such as decreased gastrointestinal motility, delayed gastric and intestinal emptying, reduction of gastric acid secretion, and increased mucous secretion. During late pregnancy, an increase in alveolar ventilation as well as tidal volume is observed (Alaily and Caroll 1978), which may enhance the pulmonary absorption of drugs given by inhalation. In addition, the increase in venous pressure in the lower limbs could alter the absorption rate of drugs administered intramuscularly.

Distribution. The physical changes related to pregnancy which may modify the distribution of a drug and/or its metabolites include the increase in total body water (both intra- and extra-vascular), large accumulation of body fat, the decrease in drug binding to plasma proteins (albumin), and profound hemodynamic changes.

Metabolism. Maternal drug biotransformation could be a major determinant of the therapeutic and/or fetotoxic effect(s) of a drug. Increased hepatic microsomal production of a diol (via epoxide) metabolite has been found for phenytoin during early pregnancy (Blake et al. 1978). Increased plasma free fraction due to decreased albumin binding may increase the rate of metabolism. Pseudocholinesterase concentrations fall during pregnancy and may result in an impaired ability to hydrolyze the muscle relaxant succinylcholine. However, the rates of maternal drug biotransformation may vary as a function of gestational age and may be affected differently in various organs of the same animal. The relative rates of bioactivating versus inactivating reactions for any given substrate may also be affected by pregnancy. Most studies on the effects of pregnancy on rates of drug biotransformation have been performed using in vitro enzyme preparations. Therefore, further studies need to be carried out in various species of whole animal to demonstrate the pregnancy-dependent differences in drug biotransforming enzyme systems.

Excretion. Pregnancy-dependent increases in renal plasma flow and glomerular filtration rate would increase the kidney excretion rates of drug and/or its metabolites. Decreases in plasma albumin binding may also increase the rate of renal excretion of the unbound drug or/and its metabolites. Biliary excretion of the injected dye sulfobromophthalein was found to decrease during pregnancy (Tindall 1975). Whether the biliary excretion of other foreign chemicals would be similarly affected is unknown. Pulmonary excretion of gases and volatile substances would be increased due to increased respiratory rate, tidal volume, and minute volume.

Placental Factors

Placental Transfer. The placental transfer of a compound may be influenced by the following factors: blood flow rates of the placental circulation--uterine and umbilical; lipid solubility of the compound and its degree of ionization in the maternal and fetal circulations; molecular weight of the compound; protein binding of the compound in the maternal and fetal plasma; and the stage of development of the placenta. Mirkin and Singh (1976) have provided a thorough review of this subject.

Placental Metabolism. Placental metabolism of drugs and foreign chemicals has been thoroughly reviewed by Juchau (1976). The therapeutic significance of drug biotransformation in the placenta remains to be defined under in vivo conditions. However, fetotoxic effects of drugs or foreign chemicals may be induced by placental metabolism and this area of research requires further investigation (Goodman et al. 1982).

Fetal Factors

Distribution. Nearly all drugs distribute to various tissues after entry into the fetus. The distribution is influenced by the altered permeability of specific membranes, or by the content of total body water and lipids in the fetus, and the altered distribution of fetal circulation. A variable proportion of umbilical venous blood will bypass the liver and an alteration in hepatic blood flow would occur. Some drugs accumulate in the amniotic fluid via urinary excretion or by exchange across the nonkeratinized fetal skin or across the chorioamnion or respiratory epithelium. Recycling of drugs between the fetus and amniotic fluid may occur through fetal swallowing of amniotic fluid.

Metabolism. Fetal drug metabolism has been extensively investigated using in vitro enzyme preparations. Experiments under in vivo conditions are essential to determine the role of fetal metabolism in eliciting the therapeutic and fetotoxic effects of drugs in the fetus. The developmental aspects of drug metabolizing enzymes at different gestational ages should also be investigated in utero.

Excretion. Renal function in the fetus is underdeveloped. Both glomerular filtration rate and renal plasma flow rate are lower on a body weight basis; tubular secretion of organic compounds is restricted. This results in prolonged elimination half-life for polar, water soluble compounds in the fetal circulation.

CONCLUSION

The therapeutic and toxicologic effects of drug exposure to the fetus are governed by a combination of factors which modify the pharmacokinetics of drugs and metabolites in the mother, placenta, and fetus. The role of pharmacokinetic studies in prenatal pharmacology and toxicology is, therefore, to characterize the essential pharmacokinetic parameters that determine the therapeutic benefits or/and fetotoxic risks of drug use during pregnancy. Well-designed and properly conducted pharmacokinetic experiments will provide valuable information on drug disposition in the maternal-placental-fetal unit.

A systematic pharmacokinetic study of drug and metabolite disposition in the maternal-placental-fetal unit was described. The model drug, acetaminophen, was found to be transferred across the placenta via passive diffusion into the fetal circulation and metabolized in the fetus to the glucuronide and sulfate conjugates. Transplacental clearances of acetaminophen from the maternal and fetal circulation were found to be equivalent. No placental metabolism of acetaminophen was observed. No transplacental transfer of acetaminophen conjugates was detected. Both acetaminophen glucuronide and sulfate are predominantly eliminated from the plasma through renal excretion via glomerular filtration in the fetal kidney and by renal tubular secretion and glomerular filtration in the maternal kidney. Knowing the disposition of the conjugates, we could then determine the conjugation activities in the ewes and in the fetal lambs in utero. Glucuronidation and sulfation activities are much lower in the fetal lambs than those in the ewes. Therefore, both conjugation pathways could possibly be saturated in the fetus should a large dose of acetaminophen be taken by the mother. If a reactive metabolite of acetaminophen could be formed in the fetus, saturation of the conjugation pathways could lead to toxic effects in the fetus. Further studies are required to characterize the oxidative metabolism and glutathione conjugation pathways in the fetus in utero before the potential toxicity of acetaminophen to the fetus can be assessed.

REFERENCES

Alaily, A.B., and Caroll, K.B. Pulmonary ventilation in pregnancy. Br J Obstet Gynaecol 85:518-524, 1978.

Amon, I., and Amon, K. Zum Ubertritt von Arzneimitteln in das Fruchtwasser. Zentralb Gynakol 98:961-969, 1976.

Aranda, J.V., and Stern, L. Clinical aspects of developmental pharmacology and toxicology. Pharmacol Ther 20:1-51, 1983.

Benet, L.Z. Pharmacokinetics: Basic principles and its use as a tool in drug metabolism. In: Mitchell, J.R., and Horning, M.G., eds. Drug Metabolism and Drug Toxicity. New York: Raven Press, 1984. pp. 199-211.

Blake, D.A.; Collins, J.M.; Mayasaki, B.C.; and Cohen, F. Influence of pregnancy and folic acid on phenytoin metabolism by rat liver microsomes. Drug Metab Dispos 6:246-250, 1978.

Bogaert, M.C., and Thiery, M. Pharmacokinetics and pregnancy. Eur J Obstet Gynecol Reprod Biol 16:229-235, 1983.

Carson, G.D.; Bolla, J.D.; and Challis, J.R.G. The availability of cortisol in amniotic fluid to the fetus and chorionic and amniotic membranes. Endocrinology 104:1053-1058, 1979.

Dawes, G.S. Breathing and rapid-eye movement sleep before birth. In: Comline, R.S.; Cross, K.W.; Dawes, G.S.; and Nathanielsz, P.W., eds. Fetal and Neonatal Physiology. Cambridge: Cambridge Press, 1973. pp. 49-62.

Dutton, G.J., and Leakey, J.E.A. The perinatal development of drug metabolizing enzymes. Prog Drug Res 25:189-273, 1982.

Gabrielsson, J.L., and Paalzow, L.K. A physiological pharmacokinetic model for morphine disposition in the pregnant rat. J Pharmacokinet Biopharm 11:147-163, 1983.

Gillette, J.R. Factors that affect drug concentrations in maternal plasma. In: Wilson, J.G., and Fraser, F.C., eds. Handbook of Teratology. New York: Plenum Press, 1977. pp. 35-78.

Goodman, D.R.; James, R.C.; and Harson, R.D. Placental toxicology. Food Chem Toxicol 20:123-128, 1982.

Juchau, M.R. Drug biotransformation reactions in the placenta. In: Mirkin, B.L., ed. Perinatal Pharmacology and Therapeutics. New York: Academic Press, 1976. pp.71-118.

Juchau, M.R., and Faustman-Watts, E. Pharmacokinetic considerations in the maternal-placental-fetal unit. Clin Obstet Gynaecol 26:379-390, 1983.

Krauer, B., and Krauer, F. Drug kinetics in pregnancy. Clin Pharmacokinet 2:167-181, 1977.

Krauer, B.; Krauer, F.; and Hytten, F.E. Drug disposition and pharmacokinetics in the maternal-placental-fetal unit. Pharmacol Ther 10:301-328, 1980.

Levy, G., and Hayton, W.L. Pharmacokinetic aspects of placental drug transfer. In: Boreus, L.O., ed. Fetal Pharmacology. New York: Raven Press, 1973. pp.29-40.

Lucier, G.W.; Lui, E.M.K.; and Lamartiniere, C.A. Metabolic activation/deactivation reactions during perinatal development. Environ Health Perspect 29:7-16, 1979.

Mellor, D.J. Investigations of fluid spaces of the sheep conceptus. In: Nathanielsz, P.W., ed. Animal Models in Fetal Medicine. Amsterdam: Elsevier/North Holland Biomedical Press, 1980. pp.59-106.

Mirkin, B.L., and Singh, S. Placental transfer of pharmacologically active molecules. In: Mirkin, B.L., ed. Perinatal Pharmacology and Therapeutics. New York: Academic Press, 1976. pp. 1-69.

Nau, H., and Liddiard, C. Placental transfer of drugs during early human pregnancy. In: Merker, H.J.; Nau, H.; and Langman, J., eds. Role of Pharmacokinetics in Prenatal Pharmacology and Prenatal Toxicology. Stuttgart: Georg Thieme Publishers, 1978. pp. 465-481.

Pelkonen, O. Biotransformation of xenobiotics in the fetus. Pharmacol Ther 10:261-281, 1980.

Rajchgot, P., and MacLeod, S. Perinatal pharmacology. Prog Clin Biol Res 135:3-23, 1983.

Rudolph, A.M., and Heymann, M.A. Methods for studying the circulation of the fetus in utero. In: Nathanielsz, P. W., ed. Animal Models in Fetal Medicine. Amsterdam: Elsevier/North Holland Biomedical Press, 1980. pp. 1-57.

Seeds, A.E. Basic concepts of maternal-fetal amniotic fluid exchange. Pediatr Clin North Am 28:231-240, 1981.

Szeto, H.H. Pharmacokinetics in the ovine maternal-fetal unit. Annu Rev Pharmacol Toxicol 2:221-243, 1982.

Szeto, H.H.; Umans, J.G.; and Rubinow, S.I. The contribution of transplacental clearances and fetal clearance to drug disposition in the ovine maternal-fetal unit. Drug Metab Dispos 10:382-386, 1982.

Tindall, V.R. The liver in pregnancy. Clin Obstet Gynaecol 2:441-462, 1975.

Wang, L.H.; Rudolph, A.M.; and Benet, L.Z. Acetaminophen disposition in adult, neonatal and fetal sheep (abstr.) APHA Acad Pharm Sci 13(1):94, 1983.

Wang, L.H.; Rudolph, A.M.; and Benet, L.Z. The distribution and fate of acetaminophen conjugates in fetal lambs in utero. Submitted to J Pharmacol Exp Ther, 1985a.

Wang, L. H.; Rudolph, A.M.; and Benet, L.Z. Pharmacokinetic studies of the disposition of acetaminophen in the sheep maternal-placental-fetal unit. Submitted to J Pharmacol Exp Ther, 1985b.

ACKNOWLEDGMENTS

This work was supported in part by National Institute of General Medical Sciences center grant GM26691. During the course of this work, L.H. Wang was the recipient of a Chancellor's Graduate Research Fellowship at the University of California, San Francisco.

AUTHORS

Laurene H. Wang, B.S., M.S.
Graduate Research Fellow
Department of Pharmacy
School of Pharmacy
University of California
San Francisco, California 94143.

Abraham M. Rudolph, M.D.
Professor of Pediatrics, Physiology, and Obstetrics,
Gynecology and Reproduction Sciences
School of Medicine
University of California
San Francisco, California 94143

Leslie Z. Benet, Ph.D.
Professor and Chairman
Department of Pharmacy
School of Pharmacy
University of California
San Francisco, California 94143

The Pharmacodynamics of Prenatal Chemical Exposure

Richard K. Miller and Carol K. Kellogg

Pregnancy represents a unique time in the life cycle of a species. It is a collage of interacting and interdependent variables in the mother, conceptus, and placenta--modifying all three during the course of gestation in mammals. If one superimposes the introduction of a chemical in this complex milieu, the number of interactions relating to the distribution, metabolism, and effects of such an agent in mother and conceptus can be considerable.

Substantial interest has recently been focused in three major areas of developmental investigations which relate to: (1) the ability of chemicals to be metabolized to toxic products which may then produce their effects in either mother and/or conceptus; (2) specific interactions with developing processes, e.g., cell-cell interactions necessary for appropriate organ development, or receptor-specific responses; and (3) organ-specific responses leading to lethality, or reduced functional or structural capacity, e.g., the central nervous system (CNS), reproductive system, and placenta.

No single set of experimental tools can be applied to explore such questions. Most often a comprehensive evaluation of the distribution, metabolism, and interactions of a compound, whether drug or environmental chemical, must be completed for both mother and conceptus before any understanding of mechanistic actions can be established. These are common recommendations for or from a pharmacologist or toxicologist; however, these principles are often not considered critical or widely appreciated by teratologists, obstetricians, or pediatricians. Other clinicians not devoted to studies in developmental pharmacology or toxicology do not appreciate the fact that the conceptus can be a separately functioning organism from a pharmacological point of view and, therefore, these investigators are content with extrapolating observations of drug distribution, metabolism, and interaction from the nonpregnant adult, and applying them directly to the pregnant patient. This fallacy must be eliminated forever and in its place must be imprinted the following:

1. There are dramatic and continuing changes in the physiology and biochemistry of pregnancy, which include both mother and conceptus and do persist throughout the entire course of gestation.

2. There are two entirely separate and distinct genomes existing in the same organism (mother).

3. There are two separate and distinct blood supplies with a unique interface, the trophoblast.

4. There is rapid and selective growth of specific cell types in the conceptus at particular stages of gestation.

5. There are direct and indirect interactions among mother, embryo/fetus, and placenta.

With such sensitivity to basic principles of pharmacology and toxicology, it is possible to begin to assess the reasons by which certain responses in the pregnant female may differ from that of the nonpregnant female, and equally important why the conceptus (whether embryo, fetus, or placenta) may respond differently at one time from another time in its life cycle (figure 1). Yet, to evaluate the effects of chemical exposure during pregnancy, one must consider not only the immediate impact of such exposure on those cells, organs, or systems, but rather the impact on the total development and life of the mother and conceptus. How persistent or transient are the effects? Are these effects due to the presence of the chemical at the time of testing or are these effects the result of permanent alterations in system function without the persistence of the agent at the time of testing? Does the conceptus have mechanisms to guard itself against such chemical invasions or is it at the mercy and benevolence of the mother to protect and sustain the growth and development of the conceptus?

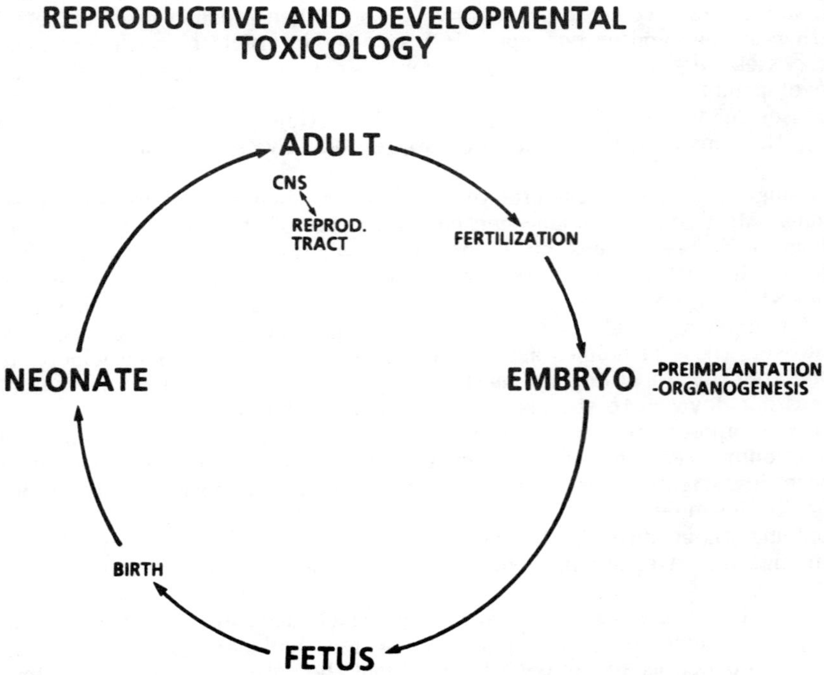

FIGURE 1. The continuum of perinatal pharmacology and toxicology.

These questions of pharmacodynamics will be addressed by evaluating two classes of compounds and organ systems: (1) Heavy metal toxicity and placental function; and (2) ataratics and CNS function. Through these examples, specificity and selectivity of chemical distribution in mother and conceptus as well as organs/cells will be explored with an emphasis on the selectivity of chemical response in mother and conceptus either in utero or as an adult.

Before investigating specific examples, please refer to figure 2 which presents a general review of the principal variables for consideration during pregnancy for the mother, placenta, and conceptus. These factors will be discussed in the following pages only as they relate to the specific examples presented. For a detailed discussion of these factors, the reader is referred to Miller et al. (1976) and Miller (1983).

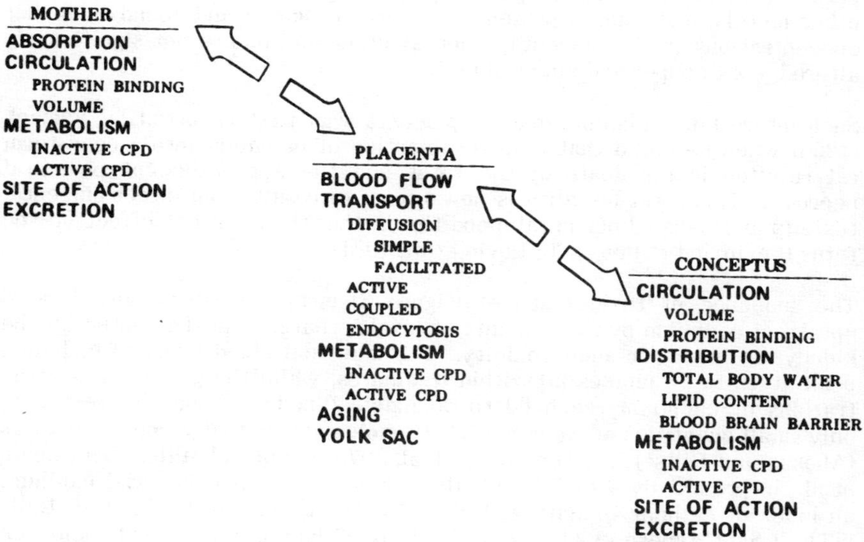

FIGURE 2. Biochemical and physiological consideration in prenatal exposure to chemicals (from Miller 1983. Copyright 1983, Alan R. Liss, Inc.)

HEAVY METAL TOXICITY AND PLACENTAL FUNCTION

Heavy metals, in particular lead, mercury, and cadmium, are associated with birth defects and alterations in growth (cf. Clarkson et al. 1983). The usual exposure to such metals is considered to be occupational or environmental (in air, water, or food); however, it is becoming apparent that substance abuse in the form of cigarette smoking can result in the accumulation of cadmium within the body. One organ which appears to concentrate these metals is the placenta (cf. Miller and Shaikh 1983). The concentration of these metals in the human placenta has been correlated with such environmental and occupational exposures (Clark 1977; Hubermont et al. 1978; Lauwerys et al. 1978; Khera et al. 1980).

Placentae from many regions of the world have been evaluated for the concentration of cadmium (cf. Miller and Shaikh 1983). Unfortunately, there is wide variation within any given locale for the actual levels of cadmium when compared with lead or mercury. As noted above, the reason for such variation is attributed to the personal habits of the individuals as correlated with the amount of cigarette smoking. Studies in multiple laboratories and geographical regions have confirmed this association between cigarette smoking and placental concentration of cadmium (table 1). It has been proposed that the placenta be an exposure index for selected environmental chemicals. Yet, such questions as level of risk, dose-response relationships, and actual form of the metals have not been investigated extensively.

Cadmium rapidly appears in the blood when a person inhales it via cigarette smoke. In our laboratory, we have noted cadmium levels between 4 and 8 ng/ml in blood after smoking a single cigarette. Thus, besides the carbon monoxide, nicotine, cyanide, polycyclic aromatic hydrocarbons, and other metals, cadmium is present in cigarette smoke and found in higher concentrations in the placenta, whereas other metals are not significantly altered, e.g., copper and zinc (table 1).

Such interest in cadmium and the placenta was first reported by Parizek (1964) when he noted that a single injection of cadmium into a near-term rat resulted in the death of the fetus and the appearance of placental necrosis. This fetal lethality is now known to result from direct placental toxicity and reduced placental blood flow rather than a direct effect on the fetus (Levin and Miller 1980; Levin et al. 1981).

The sequence of toxic response (figure 3) is apparently an initial rapid uptake of cadmium by the placenta at levels greater than that noted by the kidney, an index for adult toxicity. The maternal blood levels of cadmium peak at 18 to 20 nmoles/ml within 5 minutes, while the placental concentrations of cadmium reach 60 to 90 nmoles/gm by 1 hour. Interestingly, only small quantities of cadmium (<0.1 nmoles/gm) actually enter the fetus (Ahokas and Dilts 1979; Sonawane et al. 1975; Levin and Miller 1980; Levin et al., in press). By 4 to 6 hours, there is a rise in mitochondrial calcium, an index of cellular toxicity and ultrastructural damage (Levin et al. 1981, 1983; di Sant'Agnese et al. 1983). By 10 to 12 hours, a 5 percent incidence of fetal death, a low incidence of histologic placental necrosis, and a 25 percent reduction <u>in utero</u> placental blood flow were all observed (Levin and Miller 1981). By 18 hours, all of these observations increased substantially. Recently, cadmium administration during late gestation in rodents reduced the placental transfer of cobalamin while not significantly altering neutral amino acid transfer (Danielsson and Dencker 1984). Such dramatic changes indicate the potential for a single dose of cadmium administered near term in the rat to produce placental toxicity with resultant fetal lethality.

Wolkowski (1974) hypothesized that it is not cadmium which produces the placental toxicity, but rather metallothionein, a 10,000 dalton protein which binds cadmium and other metals. Metallothionein is a known nephrotoxin. However, metallothionein injected intravenously into the mother did not produce fetal death, but did produce nephrotoxicity. While blood levels of cadmium dropped from 18 nmoles/ml to 1 nmole/ml, the content of cadmium in the placenta did not increase comparably (Plautz et al. 1980; Levin et al. 1981).

TABLE 1. Placental Levels of Cadmium, Copper, and Zinc in Women Who Do or Do Not Smoke

Location	No.	Cadmium ng/g	Copper ug/g	Zinc ug/g	Reference
Belgium					
Nonsmoker	333	12.5 ± 8.6	--	--	Roels et al. 1978
Smoker	109	15.7 ± 9.2*	--	--	
Netherlands					
Nonsmoker	31	8.2 ± 3.2	--	--	Van Hattum et al. 1981
Smoker	30	10.6 ± 5.2*	--	--	
Rochester, NY					
Nonsmoker	18	4.3 ± 2.8	11.76 ± 0.65	1.24 ± 0.10	Miller and Gardner 1981
Smoker	24	19.2 ± 4.6*	11.94 ± 0.64	1.36 ± 0.08	
Cleveland, Ohio					
Nonsmoker	31	13.7 ± 6.4	--	--	Kuhnert et al. 1982
Smoker	44	18.1 ± 7.3*	--	--	

*Significantly different at least at ($P < 0.05$).

The placenta levels of cadmium in the human study were similar to levels found in the rodent (Wier et al. 1983b), and the resultant functions of the placenta during prolonged perfusion with complete transfusions every 4 hours were notably compromised. The fetal circuit began to lose volume (>5 ml/hr) between 8 to 10 hours of perfusion; the production, tissue content, and perfusate levels of human chorionic gonadotropin were depressed by 85 percent. Further, the stroma became edematous, Hofbauer cells were vacuolated, and subsynctiotrophoblastic vacuolization became widely apparent, as has also been noted for cycloheximide exposure (Wier et al., in press).

Therefore, besides studying the distribution, metabolism, and transfer of chemicals between the maternal and fetal circulations, the tissue content and alterations in both structure and function over periods between 12 to 16 hours can be examined to answer the question: Does a compound appear in the fetal circulation? In addition, the human question of how chemicals interact with the placenta and its circulation and function now can be studied without risk to mother or baby.

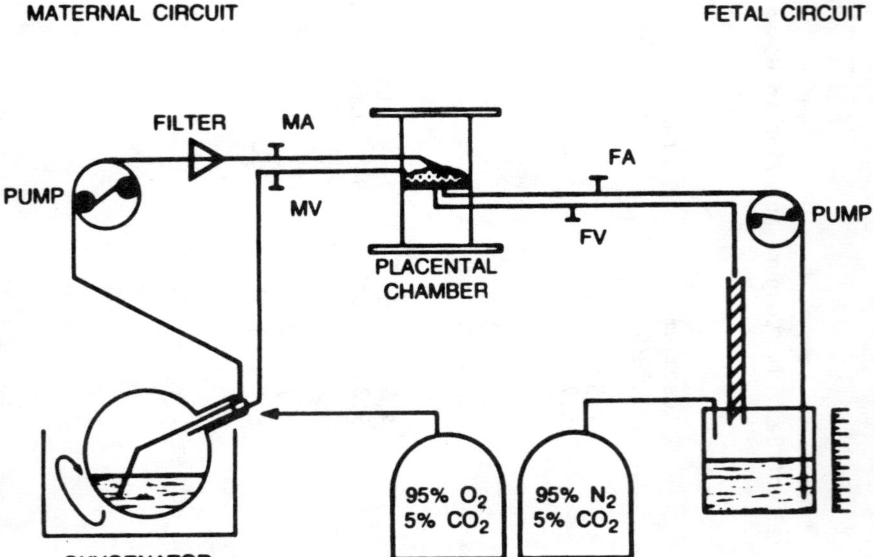

FIGURE 4. Diagram of a dual perfused recirculating human placental lobule perfusion.

The placenta, whether human or rodent, does result in chemical-induced pathology (Panigel 1981; Miller and Thiede 1981, 1984). It is proposed that prolonged perfusion of the human placenta under in vitro conditions may offer an opportunity for assessing not only transfer and metabolism by human fetal tissue-trophoblast but also the potential for determining the toxicity of both drugs and environmental chemicals. The transfer and metabolism of diazepam has been studied under short-term perfusion conditions for the human placenta (Guerre-Milo et al. 1982). It was found that the degree of plasma binding by diazepam and other benzodiazepines did alter the placental transfer of these ataratics.

It is apparent that this dose of cadmium, which results in placental toxicity in the rat, is greater than the levels in placentae from cigarette smokers (table 1). A dose-response relationship for different species, including man, presents multiple difficulties in gathering these epidemiologic data following acute exposure.

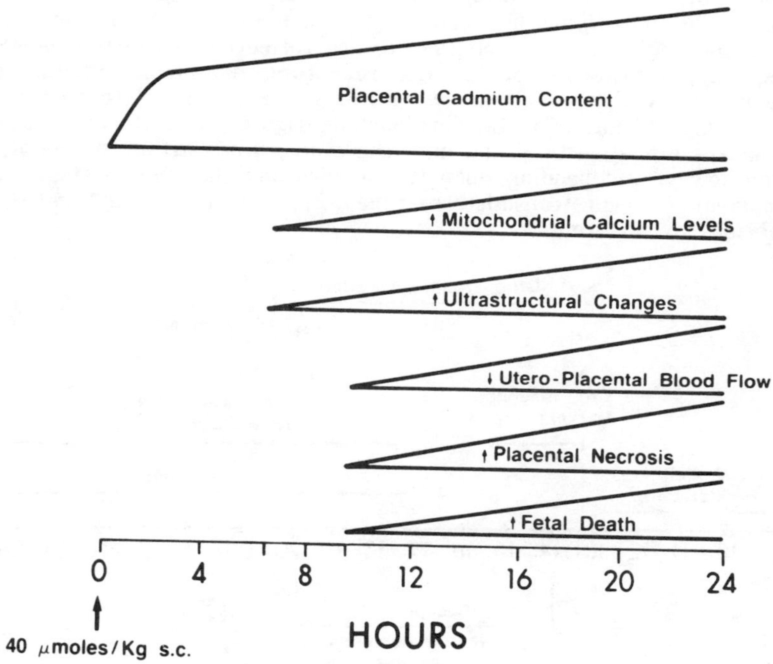

FIGURE 3. Sequence of observed responses in the near-term pregnant rat following a single subcutaneous administration of 40 umoles/kg of cadmium chloride. The lines represent a relative change in structure, concentration, or function without direct comparisons to absolute values among the variables measured. This figure summarizes the observations reported by Levin and Miller (1980, 1981), Levin et al. (1981, 1983, in press), and Miller et al. (1983).

To compare the species similarities and differences, an in vitro human placental system that allows for 12-hour perfusion was developed (Miller et al. 1985) to explore the direct toxicity of cadmium on the human placenta (figure 4). This perfusion system is based on the model developed by Panigel (1962) and Schneider et al. (1972). In the rat, following a subcutaneous dose of cadmium chloride of 40 nmoles/kg, the plasma levels of cadmium were 18 nmoles/ml at 5 minutes and 1 nmole/ml after 1 to 2 hours (Levin et al., in press). These kinetics for cadmium were reproduced in the in vitro human placental perfusion where initial doses were either 10 or 100 nmoles/ml. In particular, little cadmium passed to the fetal circulation in either the rat or human study, while the placenta concentrated cadmium in excess of 100 nmoles/gm.

PRENATAL DIAZEPAM AND POSTNATAL FUNCTION

The developing brain can be permanently altered by drugs which have only acute or transient effects on the adult nervous system. Such permanent alterations in CNS function following exposure of chemicals to the developing brain may be different from those effects noted following adult therapy. The underlying mechanisms for such differences in responses between the adult and developing brains are reflected in the sequence of events, e.g., appearance of specific receptors, neurotransmitters, cell types, and cell-cell interactions, which are spatially related to particular stages of in utero and neonatal development (figure 5). In the adult, these relationships are all established and, therefore, drugs affect a complete system; however, depending upon the species and the growth stage, the development of neurotransmitters, receptors, cell types, and cell-cell interactions are different.

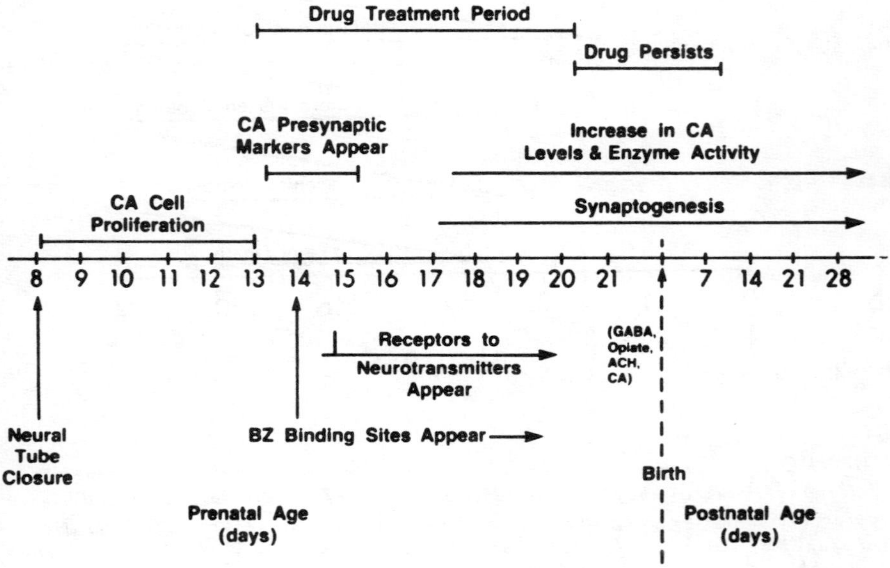

FIGURE 5. Prenatal exposure of diazepam to rats during the last week of gestation and the persistence of the drug in the brains of the progeny as related to developmental events in the fetal and neonatal brains. Prenatal and postnatal age are indicated on the horizontal line. Late gestation in the rat is characterized by rapid neuronal proliferation and differentiation as well as by the beginning of synaptic formation. Specific receptors for drugs and transmitters begin appearing during this period. Abbreviations: CA = catecholamine, BZ = benzodiazepine, ACh = acetylcholine, GABA = gamma aminobutyric acid.

Even though organogenesis (embryogenesis) in both man and rat can be compared, the rapid development of the rat suggests that even single exposure to a drug may be equivalent to multiple exposures in man.

Malformations of the CNS, such as spina bifida and anecephaly, are developmental anomalies due to the effects of an agent directly on the neural tube during embryogenesis. However, during this time of gestation, the specific receptors and neurotransmitters apparently are not present or functional. Therefore, the specificity of CNS drug action on the developing CNS would be predominant when the appearance of these specific neurochemical processes are present. Such development is seen from approximately the 10th week in the human and day 10 or 11 in the rat. Therefore, for a number of functional defects the fetal period may be the most susceptible time in the life cycle.

Is there though a comparison between the human and the rodent when one is assessing behavior, function, and the effects of drugs? The answer must be an emphatic yes with the caveat that one is examining mechanisms of action and, therefore, the potential species differences are adequately considered before conclusions are drawn. Such examinations must include pharmacokinetics/dynamics, developmental sequences, intercurrent disease, and the exact timing of the drug exposures.

The question of whether drugs or environmental chemicals do alter postnatal function has been reviewed extensively by other investigators (Rodier 1980; Vorhees and Butcher 1982; Hutchings, in press). Many psychoactive agents act on specific mechanisms of neurotransmitter function, e.g., transmitter receptors, reuptake sites, synthesizing enzymes, or release mechanisms. However, how specifically, selectively, and extensively can a drug modify postnatal function following in utero drug exposure has not been resolved.

Diazepam, a minor tranquilizer, has been investigated in animals to explore these questions because of the variety of regulatory dysfunctions noted in the human neonate whose mother had taken diazepam during pregnancy (Scher et al. 1972; Cree et al. 1973; Safra and Oakley 1978; Rementeria and Bhatt 1982). Even maternal stress itself induces functional impairments in the progeny (Ward 1972). Such functional alterations due to maternal stress have been prevented by concurrent diazepam therapy during pregnancy (Barlow et al. 1979). However, does such therapy represent a specific and permanent interaction within the developing brain?

Diazepam, when administered between days 13 to 20 of gestation in the rat (where gestation is 21 to 22 days), can modify a number of behavioral endpoints during postnatal development and in adult life, i.e., startle response, auditory temporal resolution, and coping with stress, without significantly altering more general behaviors (Kellogg et al. 1980, 1983b; Simmons et al. 1984b). These specific behavioral changes are related to maternal doses of diazepam (1 to 10 mg/kg). Such selectivity in response indicates a specific mechanistic interaction. Previous investigations have characterized a benzodiazepine receptor in the adult which interacts with both the GABAminergic and catecholaminergic neurons (cf. Gee et al. 1984).

These alterations in adult behavior following prenatal exposure to diazepam are not related to the continued presence of diazepam into adult life since the pups were fostered to control mothers at birth and diazepam was undetectable in the neonatal brain or other tissues by day 20 (table 2).

TABLE 2. The Distribution of Diazepam and its Metabolites in Selected Tissues of the Mother and Neonates Following *In Utero* Administration of 2.5 mg/kg of ^{14}C-Diazepam Between Days 13 to 20 of Gestation (Simmons et al. 1983).

	Total Diazepam/Metabolites in Selected Tissues pmoles/100mg				Proportion of Diazepam and Metabolites in Brain			
	Plasma	Liver	Heart	Brain	Diazepam	N-desmethyl-diazepam	Oxazepam	Glucuronide
Maternal	3.7±0.5	55.8±7.7	20.1±1.4	3.4±0.3	24±5%	28±4%	0%	49±2%
Neonatal 0	ND	7.8±0.9	6.3±0.5	3.2±0.3	24±9%	25±9%	0%	52±4%
Neonatal 10	ND	ND	ND	3.4±0.3	19±8%	39±9%	12±6%	32±5%
Neonatal 20	ND	ND	ND	ND	ND	ND	ND	ND

ND - not detectable

Thus, persistent functional alterations are present in the adult progeny following only prenatal exposure to diazepam, even though the drug is no longer present.

A mechanistic evaluation of these aberrant behaviors was initiated to determine: (1) the relationship to stress, (2) the neurochemical impairments (GABA, GAD, norepinephrine), (3) regional specificity of such changes, and (4) receptor specificity. Since sensory perception was altered by prenatal exposure to diazepam, does diazepam permanently alter the ability of the offspring to respond to stress? Following restraint stress, the adult control progeny demonstrated the typical response for plasma corticosterone changes to such stress (figure 6). However, prenatal exposure to diazepam prevents the surges in this hormone following such stress. Thus, the ability of these animals treated <u>in utero</u> with diazepam to respond normally to stress was impaired.

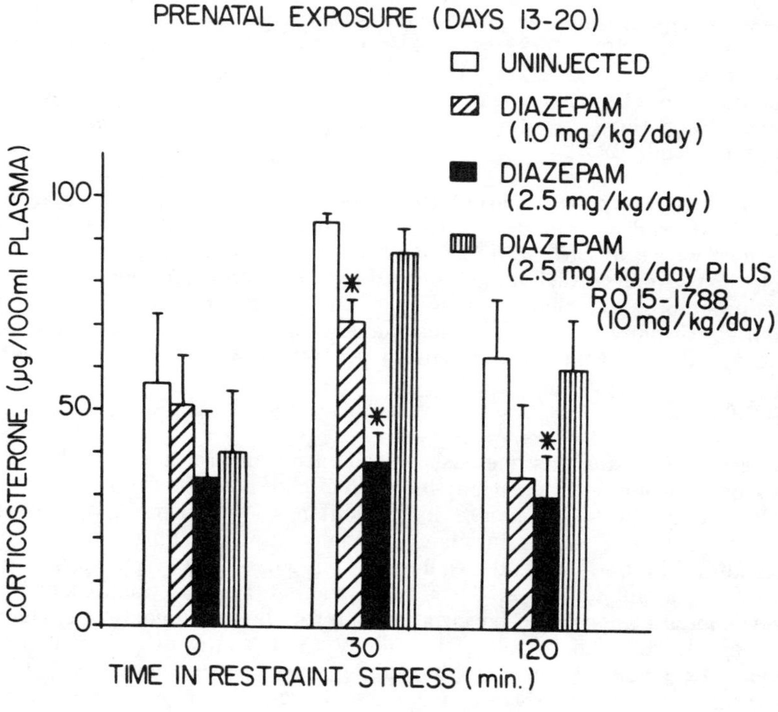

FIGURE 6. Plasma levels of corticosterone in 90-day-old rat progeny under basal conditions and following 30 or 120 minutes of restraint stress. The stressor was restraint stress, which was induced by placing the animal in a small plastic restraint cage located in a brightly lighted room for specific time intervals. Asterisk denotes a significant difference ($p < 0.05$) from controls at each individual time period as determined by Student's -t-test. Corticosterone was measured by a specific radioimmunoassay using dog corticosterone binding globulin as the antibody (from Simmons et al. 1984b, Copyright 1984, Elsevier Science Publishers, B.V.).

Such hormonal regulation would implicate the hypothalamus in the control of these processes. Regional neurochemical determinations of GABA receptors, norepinephrine, and glutamic acid-decarboxylase demonstrated that only norepinephrine content and turnover were decreased in a dose-related manner by diazepam in the hypothalamus of the adult progeny (table 3). These alterations in norepinephrine neurons occurred when no significant changes in the number of binding sites, dissociation constant, or maximal stimulation by GABA were noted for benzodiazepine binding in newborns or adults prenatally exposed to 2.5 or 10 mg/kg/day of diazepam (Kellogg et al. 1983b).

Such selectivity of neurochemical and functional responses would be consistent with a specific activation mechanism. Fortunately, a benzodiazepine antagonist for the central binding sites (RO15-1788) is available. RO15-1788 does not appear to have agonist activity but rather blocks diazepam at the receptor (Gee et al. 1984). To determine whether the benzodiazepine receptor is involved in the production of these functional impairments, RO15-1788 was coadministered to the pregnant dam with diazepam. Prenatal RO15-1788 blocked the inhibitory effects of prenatal diazepam on the stress-induced corticosterone surge (figure 6) and the content and turnover of norepinephrine in the hypothalamus of the adult progeny (table 4).

Thus, it is becoming apparent that specific CNS functions may be permanently altered by prenatal exposures to drugs which have selective interactions with the CNS while many other functions may appear normal. Such selectivity and specificity of interactions between drug and regions of the brain demonstrate that what may be a transient yet specific effect in the adult brain may be just as selective and specific--receptor mediated--in the developing brain with a resultant permanent alteration.

CONCLUSION

Cigarette smoking has been associated with small for gestation age infants, postnatal growth retardation, induction of mixed function oxidases, and other delays in development. In particular, cadmium has been documented to be at higher levels in placentae of cigarette smokers than in non-smokers. In both animal studies and in vitro human placenta perfusion studies, cadmium has been found to be placental toxic. Such specificity for the placenta appears to be greater than for the organ commonly thought to represent cadmium toxicity, the kidney. Yet, many other constituents of cigarette smoke do modify the capacity of the conceptus, e.g., nicotine affects uterine blood flow, placental transport of nutrients, and fetal breathing; polycyclic aromatic hydrocarbons affect fetal and placental metabolism of xenobiotics (cf. Sastry et al. 1983; Juchau 1980, 1982, this volume; Pelkonen, 1980; Miller et al., 1983).

The metabolism of drugs and environmental chemicals has been implicated in their developmental toxicity, e.g., benzo(a)pyrene (Nebert 1981), phenytoin (Martz et al. 1977), cyclophosphamide (Manson and Smith 1977; Kitchin et al. 1981), diethylstilbestrol (cf. Metzler 1984), and thalidomide (Gordon et al. 1981). Such formation of reactive intermediates may mean that the parent compound has different therapeutic effects compared with

TABLE 3. Kinetics of Norepinephrine Turnover in Adult Hypothalamus in Rats Exposed *In Utero* to Diazepam Between Days 13 to 20 of Gestation (Simmons et al. 1984a).

Prenatal exposure days 13-20	No.	NE levels (ng/g)	Turnover rate (ng/g/h)	Turnover rate constant(h^{-1})	Turnover time (h)	Linear regression coefficient
Uninjected	23	1895 ± 221	322	0.17 ± 0.01	5.9	0.89
Vehicle	21	1688 ± 108	388	0.23 ± 0.02*	4.4	0.88
Diazepam 1.0 mg/kg	20	1304 ± 130*	241	0.18 ± 0.02	5.6	0.81
Diazepam 2.5 mg/kg	21	1238 ± 110*	112	0.09 ± 0.02	11.1	0.92
Diazepam 10 mg/kg	17	657 ± 108*	46	0.07 ± 0.02*	14.3	0.90

*Significantly different from control value, $P < 0.05$.
Mean ± S.E.M.
No.= number of animals

TABLE 4. Kinetics of Norepinephrine Turnover in the Adult Hypothalamus: Effect of Prenatal Exposure to a Benzodiazepine Antagonist (Simmons et al. 1984a).

Prenatal exposure days 13-20	NO.	NE levels (ng/g)	Turnover rate (ng/g/h)	Turnover rate constant (h^{-1})	Turnover time (h)	Linear regression coefficient
Uninjected	15	1719 ± 138	292	0.17 ± 0.01	5.9	0.88
RO-1788 10 mg/kg	15	1695 ± 152	278	0.16 ± 0.02	6.1	0.82
RO-1788 10 mg/kg & Diazepam 2.5 mg/kg	15	1662 ± 133	288	0.17 ± 0.01	5.8	0.92
Diazepam 2.5 mg/kg	15	1298 ± 112*	117	0.09 ± 0.01*	11.1	0.90

*Significantly different from control value, $P < 0.05$.
No. = number of animals
Mean ± S.E.M.

the toxicity of their reactive metabolites (arene oxides, epoxides, phenoxyradicals). In fact, it may be the metabolic capability of the conceptus which determines the developmental toxicity of a compound and not just the maternal capabilities as demonstrated for benzo(a)pyrene metabolism by embryos in the same litter (Shum et al. 1979). Thus, the pharmacogenetics of the conceptus may partially account for why only 1 out of 10 babies have the fetal phenytoin syndrome, especially since electrophilic intermediates of phenytoin have been implicated in producing birth defects in mice (Martz et al. 1977). Thus, for some drugs, it may not be the effect of the parent compound but other effects of its metabolites.

Besides metabolism, protein binding of drugs in both mother and conceptus may be critical to the expressed toxicity. In the rodent, synthetic estrogens such as diethylstilbestrol (DES) are both carcinogenic and teratogenic at doses lower than those noted for natural estrogens, such as estradiol. Such selectivity in response, especially in the rat, relates to: (1) specific plasma binding protein for the natural estrogen, estradiol, which circulates in the fetus; (2) the rapid metabolism of estradiol; and (3) the responsiveness of the developing reproductive tract, which is substantially different from that of the adult. In the fetus, one of the primary reasons estradiol is less teratogenic than DES is that the affinity of alpha-fetoprotein for estradiol is much greater than for DES. Therefore, less estradiol is available for entry into the tissue (cf. Miller et al. 1982, in press).

Persistent and selective alterations in the CNS can be induced following exposure to low doses of diazepam during the last week of gestation in the rat. Aberrant responses to stress have been observed in the adult progeny when no trace of the drug is detectable. Yet, of greater interest is the selectivity of this prenatal diazepam exposure for reducing hypothalamic norepinephrine levels and turnover in the adult progeny and the prevention of these aberrant behavioral responses and neurochemical alterations in the hypothalamus following coadministration of a diazepam antagonist with diazepam during gestation. Thus, these examples of prenatal exposure to cadmium, DES, and diazepam demonstrate the important differences in their individual pharmacokinetics, which include distribution, metabolism, protein binding, specific tissues, and even receptor interactions.

REFERENCES

Ahokas, R.A., and Dilts, P.V. Cadmium uptake by the rat embryo as a function of gestational age. Am J Obstet Gynecol 135:219-222, 1979.

Barlow, S.M.; Knight, A.F.; and Sullivan, F.M. Prevention by diazepam of adverse effects of maternal restraint or postnatal development and learning in the rat. Teratology 19:105-110, 1979.

Cher, J.; Hailey, D.M.; and Beard, R.W. Effects of diazepam on the fetus. J Obstet Gynaecol Br Cmwlth 79:635-638, 1972.

Clark, A.R.L. Placental transfer of lead and its effect on the newborn. Postgrad Med J 55:673-678, 1977.

Clarkson, T.; Nordberg, G.; and Sager, P. Development and Reproductive Toxicity of Metals. New York: Plenum Press, 1983.

Cree, J.E.; Meyer, J.; and Hailey, D.N. Diazepam in labour: Its metabolism and effect on the clinical condition and thermogenesis of the newborn. Br Med J 4:251-255, 1973.

Danielsson, B.R. and Dencker, L. Effects of cadmium on the placental uptake and transport to the fetus of nutrients. Biol Res Pregnancy Perinatol Vol. 5:93-101, 1984.

di Sant'Agnese, P.A.; Jensen, K.; Leven, A.A.; and Miller, R.K. Placental toxicity of cadmium: An ultrastructural study. Placenta 4:149-164, 1983.

Gee, K.W.; Yamamura, S.H.; Roeske, W.R.; and Yamamura, H.I. Benzodiazepine receptor heterogeneity: possible molecular basis of functional significance. Fed Proc 43:2767-2772, 1984.

Gordon, G.B.; Spielberg, S.P.; Blake, D.A.; and Balasubramanian, V. Thalidomide teratogenesis: Evidence for toxic arene oxide metabolite. Proc Natl Acad Sci USA 78:2545-2548, 1981.

Guerre-Milo, M.; Challier, J.C.; Rey, E.; Nandakumaran, M.; Richard, M.O.; and Olive, G. Maternofetal transfer of two benzodiazepines: effect of plasma protein binding and placental uptake. Dev Pharmacol Ther 4:158-172, 1982.

Hubermont, G.; Bucket, J.P.; Roels, H.; and Lauwerys, R. Placental transfer of lead, mercury, and cadmium in women living in a rural area. Int Arch Occup Environ Health 41:117-124, 1978.

Hutchings, D.E. Prenatal drug exposure and the problems of casual inference. In: Pinkert, T.M., ed. Current Research on the Consequences of Maternal Drug Abuse. National Institute on Drug Abuse Research Monograph 59, in press.

Juchau, M.R., Drug biotransformation in the placenta. Pharmacol Ther 8:501-524, 1980.

Juchau, M.R. The role of the placenta and development toxicology, In: Snell, K., ed., Developmental Toxicology. New York: Praeger Publishers. pp. 187-210, 1982.

Kellogg, C.K.; Tervo, D.; Ison, J.; Parisi, T.; and Miller, R.K. Prenatal exposure to diazepam alters behavioral development in rats. Science 207:205-207, 1980.

Kellogg, C.; Ison, J.; and Miller, R.K. Prenatal diazepam exposure: Effects on auditory temporal resolution in rats. Psychopharmacologia 79:332-227, 1983a.

Kellogg, C.K.; Chisholm, J.; Simmons, R.D.; Ison, J.; and Miller, R.K. Neural and behavioral consequences of prenatal exposure to diazepam. Monogr Neural Sci 9:119-129, 1983b.

Khera, A.K.; Wibberley, D.G.; and Dathan, J.G. Placental and stillbirth tissue lab concentrations in occupationally exposed women. Br J Ind Med 37:394-396, 1980.

Kitchin, K.T.; Schmid, V.P.; and Sanyal, M.K. Teratogenicity of cyclophosphamide in a coupled microsomal activating/embryo culture system. Biochem Pharmacol 30:59-64, 1981.

Kuhnert, P.M.; Kuhnert, B.R.; Bottoms, S.F.; and Erhard, P. Cadmium levels in maternal blood, fetal cord blood, and placental tissues of pregnant women who smoke. Am J Obstet Gynecol 142:1021-1025, 1982.

Lauwerys, R.; Bucket, J.P.; Roels, H.; and Hubermont, G. Placental transfer of lead, mercury, cadmium, and carbon monoxide. Environ Res 15:278-289, 1978.

Levin, A.A., and Miller, R.K. Fetal toxicity of cadmium in the rat: Maternal vs. fetal injections. Teratology 22:1-6, 1980.

Levin, A.A., and Miller, R.K. Fetal toxicity of cadmium in the rat: Decreased uteroplacental blood flow. Toxicol Appl Pharmacol 58:297-306, 1981.

Levin, A.A.; Plautz, J.R.; di Sant'Agnese, P.A.; and Miller, R.K. Cadmium: Placental mechanisms of fetal toxicity. Placenta [Suppl] 3:303-318, 1981.

Levin, A.A.; Miller, R.K.; and di Sant'Agnese, P.A. Heavy metal alterations of placental function: a mechanism for the induction of fetal toxicity with cadmium in the rat. In: Clarkson, T.; Nordberg, G.; and Sager, P., eds. Reproductive and Developmental Toxicity of Metals. New York: Plenum Press, 1983. pp. 633-654.

Levin, A.A.; Kilpper, R.W.; and Miller, R.K. Organ specific kinetics of a fetal toxic injection of $CdCl_2$ in the pregnant rat. Toxicol Appl Pharmacol, in press.

Manson, J.M., and Smith, C.C. Influence on cyclophosphamide and 4-ketocyclophosphamide on mouse limb development. Teratology 15:291-300, 1977.

Martz, F.; Failinger, C., III; and Blake, D.A. Phenytoin teratogenesis: Correlation between embryopathic effect and covalent binding of putative arene oxide metabolite in gestational tissue. J Pharmacol Exp Ther 203:231-239, 1977.

Metzler, M. Mechanisms of carcinogenesis induced by diethylstilbestrol. In: Schuler, H.M., ed. Comparative Perinatal Carcinogenesis. Florida: CRC Press, 1984. pp. 137-150.

Miller, R.K. Perinatal toxicology: Its recognition and fundamentals. Am J Ind Med 4:205-244, 1983.

Miller, R.K., and Gardner, K.A. Cadmium in the human placenta: relationship to smoking. Teratology 23:51, 1981.

Miller, R.K., and Shaikh, Z., Prenatal metabolism: Metals and metallothionine, In: Clarkson, T., Nordberg, G., and Sager, P., eds. Developmental and Reproductive Toxicity of Metals. New York: Plenum Press, 1983. pp. 153-204.

Miller, R.K., and Thiede, H.A., eds. Placenta: Receptors, Pathology, and Toxicology. England: Saunders. 1981.

Miller, R.K., and Thiede, H.A., eds. Fetal Nutrition, Metabolism and Immunology: Role of the Placenta. New York: Plenum Press, 1984.

Miller, R.K.; Baggs, R.B.; and Henry, E.C. Diethylstilbestrol: its teratogenicity and carcinogenicity in animals. Cervix, in press.

Miller, R.K.; Heckmann, M.E.; and McKenzie, R.C. Diethylstilbestrol: placental transfer, metabolism, covalent binding and fetal distribution in the Wistar rat. J Pharmacol Exp Ther 220:358-365, 1982.

Miller, R.K.; Koszalka, T.R.; and Brent, R.L. Transport mechanisms for molecules across placental membranes. In: Poste, G., and Nicolson, G.L., eds. Cell Surface Reviews in Animal Development. Amsterdam: Elsevier/ North Holland Biomedical Press, 1976. pp. 145-233.

Miller, R.K.; Ng, W.W.; and Levin, A.A. The placenta: Relevance to toxicology. In: Clarkson, T.W.; Nordberg, G.; and Sager, P., eds. Reproductive and Developmental Toxicity of Metals. New York: Plenum Press, 1983. pp. 569-605.

Miller, R.K.; Wier, P.J.; Maulik, D.; and di Sant'Agnese, P.A. Human placenta in vitro: characterization during 12 hours of dual perfusion. Contrib Gynecol Obstet 13:77-84, 1985.

Nebert, D.W. Birth defects and the potential genetic differences in drug metabolism. Birth Defects 17:51-70, 1981.

Panigel, M. Placental perfusion experiments. Am J Obstet Gynecol 84:1664-1672, 1962.
Panigel, M. Placental function: Toxicology and pathology. In: Miller, R.K., and Thiede, H.A., eds. Placenta: Receptors, Pathology, and Toxicology, London: Saunders, 1981. pp. 275-288.
Parizek, J. Vascular changes at sites of oestrogen biosynthesis produced by parenteral injection of cadmium salts: The destruction of the placenta by cadmium salts. J Reprod Fertil 7:263-264, 1964.
Parizek, J. The peculiar toxicity of cadmium during pregnancy: An experimental toxemia of pregnancy induced by cadmium salts. J Reprod Fertil 9:111-112, 1965.
Pelkonen, O. Environmental influences on human fetal and placental xenobiotic metabolism. Eur J Clin Pharmacol 18:17-24, 1980.
Plautz, J.R.; Levin, A.A.; and Miller, R.K. Fetal and maternal toxicity of cadmium, metallothionein and its distribution in the pregnant Wistar rat. Teratology 26:61, 1980.
Rementeria, J., and Bhatt, K. Withdrawal symptoms in neonates from in utero exposure to diazepam. J Pediatr 90:123-126, 1982
Rodier, P. Chronology of neuron development: Animal studies and their clinical implications. Dev Med Child Neurol 22:525-545, 1980.
Roels, H.; Hubermont, G.; Buchet, J.P.; and Lauwerys, R. Placental transfer of lead, mercury, cadmium, and carbon monoxide in women. Environ Res 16:236-247, 1978.
Safra, M.J., and Oakley, G.P. Association between cleft lip with or without cleft palate in prenatal exposure to diazepam. Teratology 3:47-52, 1978.
Sastry, B.B.R.; Moore, R.D.; Barnwell, S.L.; and Rowell, P.P. Factors effecting the uptake of alpha-amino acid by human placenta villus: Acetylcholine, phospholipid, methylation, calcium, and cytoskeletal organization. Trophoblast Res 1:81-100, 1983.
Scher, J.; Hailey, D.M.; and Beard, R.W. The effects of diazepam on the fetus. J Obstet Gynaecol Br Cmwlth 79:635-638, 1972.
Schneider, H.; Panigel, M.; and Dancis, J. Transfer across the perfused human placenta of antipyrine, sodium, and leucine. Am J Obstet Gynecol 114:822-828, 1972.
Shum, S.; Jensen, N.M.; and Nebert, D.M. The murine Ah locus: In utero toxicity and teratogenesis associated with genetic differences in benzo(a)pyrene metabolism. Teratology 20:365-376, 1979.
Simmons, R.D.; Miller, R.K.; and Kellogg, C.K. Prenatal diazepam: Distribution and metabolism in perinatal rats. Teratology 28:181-188, 1983.
Simmons, R.D.; Kellogg, C.K.; and Miller, R.K. Prenatal diazepam exposure in rats: Long-lasting, receptor-mediated effects on hypothalamic norepinephrine-containing neurons. Brain Res 293:73-83, 1984a.
Simmons, R.D.; Miller, R.K.; and Kellogg, C.K. Prenatal exposure to diazepam alters central and peripheral responses to stress in adult rat offspring. Brain Res 307:39-46, 1984b.
Sonawane, B.R.; Nordberg, M.; Nordberg, G.F.; and Lucier, G.W. Placental transfer of cadmium in rats: Influence of dose and gestational age. Environ Health Perspect 28:248-249, 1975.
Van Hattum, B., and de Voogt, P. An analytical procedure for the determination of cadmium in human placentae. Int J Environ Anal Chem 10:121-133, 1981.

Vorhees, C. and Butcher, R. Behavioral Teratogenicity. In: Snell, K., ed. Developmental Toxicology. New York: Praeger Publisher, 1982. pp. 247-298.

Ward, I. Prenatal stress feminizes and demasculinizes behavior of males. Science 175:82-84, 1972.

Wier, P.J., and Miller, R.K. Oxygen transfer as an indicator of perfusion variability in the isolated human placental lobule. Contrib Gynecol Obstet 13:127-131, 1985.

Wier, P.J.; Miller, R.K.; Maulik, D.; and di Sant'Agnese, P.A. The bidirectional transport of alpha-aminoisobutyric acid by the human perfused placental lobule. Trophoblast Res 1:37-54, 1983a.

Wier, P.J.; Miller, R.K.; and Maulik, D. Transfer and accumulation of cadmium by the perfused human placental lobule. Teratology 27:83-84, 1983b.

Wier, P.J.; Miller, R.K.; Maulik, D.; and di Sant'Agnese, P.A. Cadmium toxicity in the in vitro human placenta during 12 hours of perfusion. Teratology, in press.

Wolkowski, R.M. Differential cadmium-induced embryo toxicity in two inbred strains. Teratology 10:243-262, 1974.

ACKNOWLEDGMENTS

The original work presented was supported in part by National Institutes of Health grants ES 02774, CA 22335, and MH 31850, and a research award from Hoffmann-LaRoche.

AUTHORS

Richard K. Miller, Ph.D.
Associate Professor of Obstetrics/Gynecology, and
Pharmacology/ Toxicology
Director, Division of Research
University of Rochester
School of Medicine and Dentistry, Box 668
601 Elmwood Avenue
Rochester, New York 14642,

Carol K. Kellogg, Ph.D.
Professor of Psychology and Pharmacology
University of Rochester
Rochester, New York 14620

Opioids and Development: New Lessons From Old Problems

Ian S. Zagon

OLD PROBLEMS

Human consumption of opium for religious, medicinal, social, and/or personal reasons probably dates back 6,000 years (Blum 1969; Terry and Pellens 1970; Musto 1973). An important corollary to opioid[1] utilization by pregnant women relates to the passive dependence of the fetus. Exactly how long ago this relationship was perceived is unclear. However, Hippocrates (see Martin 1893) mentions opium in connection with "uterine suffocation"; this may be a reference to opium's toxicity on the embryo and/or fetus. Clearly, by the end of the 19th century, clinical reports evidenced the unusual behavior of the fetus and the neonate passively addicted to opium. Infants with "chronic opium intoxication" were reported to exhibit excessive nervousness, rapid breathing, and convulsive movements right after birth, with death occurring within the first week of life (Terry and Pellens 1970). A review of the early literature reveals an impressive amount of information and insight into the field of perinatal opioid dependence. For example, in 1895, Bureau found that morphine could pass through the human placenta. Other workers recognized the possibilities that maternal drug addiction might influence the fetus (Sainsbury 1909), and that enough opium passed into breast milk to alleviate withdrawal (Laase 1919; Langstein 1930; Petty 1912) or to even establish drug dependency in a normal infant breast-fed by a woman who became dependent on opioids after parturition (Lichenstein 1915). The importance of therapeutic intervention by administration of morphine, heroin, or paregoric to prevent withdrawal was also well recognized (Menninger-Lerchenthal 1934) by the beginning of the 20th century. Even the long-term implications of perinatal opioid exposure were noted by these early investigators. For example, in a discussion following the presentation of a paper by Earle (1888) concerning the adverse effects of fetal opioid exposure, a number of particpants reported the association of neurobiological abnormalities in offspring (including individuals reaching adulthood) maternally exposed to opium. The incidence of perinatal exposure to opioids is difficult to gauge. Perlstein (1947) and Petty (1913) refer to the "rare" occurrence of such situations in earlier periods (up to the 1940s). However, Graham-Mulhall (1926) recorded over 800 pregnant women consuming opioids in New York during a 1-year period in the early 1900s. The type of opioid abused has changed over the years. Until the 1950s, morphine appeared to be the drug of choice, with the 1956 report by Goodfriend et al. signaling a change to heroin usage. Following Dole and Nyswander's (1965) advocation of the methadone maintenance treatment program as an alternative to heroin dependency, numerous reports have documented methadone-dependent offspring. Paralleling the change from morphine to utilization of heroin and methadone in the 1950s, a marked increase in the number of births to opioid-dependent women has been recorded. In one municipal hospital in New York City, for example, only 22 infants were born to heroin-dependent mothers from 1955 to 1959, but 26 infants were delivered during 1960 (Zelson 1975). In this same hospital, over a sixfold increase in drug-dependent babies was recorded between 1960 (1 in 164 births) and 1972 (1 in 27 births). Recent estimates (Carr 1975) place the birth rate of heroin and methadone-addicted mothers at 3,000/year in New York City alone; given that New York City has one-third to one-half of the total number of chronic heroin and methadone users in the United States (Carr 1975; Salerno 1977), one could extrapolate 6,000 to 9,000 births/year to opioid-consuming women. Carr also reports that, as of 1975, 115,000 children of mothers dependent on illegal opiates and methadone maintenance were in the New York City area. Assuming again that this number for New York City is representative of one-third to one-half of the entire United States population, one can estimate that at least 250,000 infants, children, and young adults have already been born to females consuming opioids such as methadone or heroin. Placed within the context of the average number of births in the U.S. every year (roughly 3.3 million), one can calculate that at least 1 in 1,000 births is by a mother using heroin or methadone. The incidence for this "fetal opiate syndrome" or "fetal narcotic syndrome," as it may be termed, rivals estimates for many well-known and highly publicized problems of early life, including the fetal alcohol syndrome, Down's syndrome, and neural tube defects, and it far exceeds the incidence of cancer in children aged 1 to 15 years. Assuming the population of the U.S. is 230 million, and given a population of 230,000 children already exposed perinatally to opioids, 1 in 1,000 people in the U.S. have been subjected to opioids in early life. By themselves, these numbers are significant. However, unreported use of opioids by pregnant women and the possible influence exerted by paternal opiate consumption may indicate an error of underestimation.

Clinical Observation

Even before birth the offspring of opioid-dependent women are subjected to a host of potential problems. During the course of pregnancy, the mothers of these children often encounter medical complications, including infectious diseases, nutritional deficits, and an abnormal incidence of venereal disease. Obstetrical complications include toxemia of pregnancy and intrauterine growth retardation. Additionally, spontaneous miscarriage, abortion, and stillbirths have been suspected of being higher than normal among opioid-dependent women (Salerno 1977). Many of these coassociated medical and obstetrical complications appear to be secondary to the lifestyle and habits of the pregnant addict (Perlmutter 1974), with prenatal care often being neglected. The very

483-942 0 - 85 - 3 : QL 3

fact that enrollment in the methadone program places women in touch with health professionals who encourage prenatal care has been an extremely positive feature of this program.

A decrease in birthweight of infants born to heroin-dependent mothers has been recorded (Finnegan et al. 1972; Wilson et al. 1979), with low birthweight infants often being small for gestational age. These growth delays associated with prenatal heroin do not appear to be related to inadequate maternal nutrition or prenatal care (e.g., Naeye et al. 1973). In contrast to heroin-exposed offspring, methadone-dependent neonates have higher birthweights and are of greater gestational ages, although mean weight is often less than among nondrug dependent controls (Kandall et al. 1974).

Conclusive evidence that maternal opioid dependency is related to congenital malformations has not been presented, although some incidences have been reported (e.g., Ostrea and Chavez 1979). Abrahms (1975) recorded increased chromosomal aberrations in infants exposed to heroin, but not necessarily methadone, while Chavez et al. (1979) noted an increased incidence of sudden infant death syndrome (SIDS) in opioid-exposed infants. A lower incidence and severity of neonatal jaundice is known to occur for heroin-exposed infants (Zelson et al. 1973), and premature infants of heroin-dependent mothers often demonstrate a lower incidence of respiratory distress syndrome (Glass et al. 1971).

The proportion of stillbirths and mortality in the opioid-exposed population generally appears to be increased in comparison to control data (Ostrea and Chavez 1979; Perlmutter 1967), but the higher mortality rate may not be necessarily related to the neonatal withdrawal syndrome (Ostrea and Chavez 1979). Few studies have pursued details of post-mortem examination of drug-dependent infants, although evidence from neuropathological studies (e.g., Rorke et al. 1977) suggests that, in addition to a host of nonspecific secondary gestational complications, primary and specific effects of addictive drugs on the developing nervous system occur.

Perhaps the most well-recognized sign of fetal exposure to opioids is the neonatal withdrawal syndrome, with 60 to 90% of opioid-exposed infants undergoing some degree of abstinence (Perlmutter 1974). Symptoms of withdrawal include irritability, tremors, high-pitched cry, hyperactivity, wakefulness, diarrhea, disorganized sucking reflex, respiratory alkalosis, and lacrimation, as well as hiccups, sneezing, twitching, myoclonic jerks, or seizures. Opioids reported to cause these symptoms in the neonate are heroin, methadone, meperidine, morphine, codeine, and pentazocine. The onset of symptoms may be present at birth or may begin up to 14 to 28 days after birth. This depends upon the drug the infant was exposed to *in utero* and the profile of pharmacokinetic excretion. Subacute symptoms may last for 4 to 6 months after birth (Desmond and Wilson 1975).

Depending on the severity of the withdrawal syndrome, treatment with such agents as paregoric, phenobarbital, diazepam, and chlorpromazine may be required. The period of treatment may last from a few days to several months (Zelson et al. 1970). The question of advisability of breast feeding by women on opioids has been raised. Opioids are known to be present in breast milk (Blinick et al. 1975) and numerous reports describe "addictive" effects in infants consuming opioid-containing milk (Menninger-Lerchenthal 1934). Given the permeability of the blood-brain barrier during perinatal life, and the fact that only nanogram and picogram quantities of drug are required to occupy opiate receptors, it could easily be envisioned that opioids in milk could be capable of influencing the infant.

The neurobehavioral sequelae associated with perinatal opioid exposure have been extensively reviewed by Zagon and McLaughlin (1984a). In summary, a number of highlights should be mentioned. "Classical" neurological tests (Davis and Shanks 1975) have shown opioid-exposed infants to exhibit central nervous system hyperactivity, irritability, tremors and hypertonicity, impaired nutritive sucking, vomiting, severe sleep deficit, autonomic dysfunction (vasomotor lability and diarrhea), and a lability of "states" manifested by frequent shifts between sleep and wakefulness. Hyperactivity was a persistent finding that endured through the early school age (Davis and Shanks 1975). Utilizing the Brazelton Neonatal Behavioral Assessment Scale (BNBAS), a number of investigators have tried to quantitate infant response to external stimuli, motor organization, and ability to regulate state of consciousness. These studies show an impaired ability of opioid-dependent babies to adequately organize their response to environment, with a lessened capacity to attend and react to noxious stimuli and to habituate to disturbing events (Davis and Shanks 1975). Opioid-exposed infants exhibited a depressed response decrement to light, with problems in visual and auditory orientation evident (Chasnoff et al. 1982). Using the BNBAS to decipher the specific effects of methadone on the neonate, Marcus et al. (1982) have suggested that behavioral problems in methadone infants may not be due to generalized central system irritability, but actually to neuromuscular dysfunction. Other investigators have suggested that the orientation responsiveness and excitability recorded in the BNBAS have substantial impact on caregivers' perceptions of infants, which may lead to long-term consequences for caregiver-infant interactions.

During the period of infancy, a significant decrease in quiet sleep (Schulman 1969) along with an increase (Dinges et al. 1980) or decrease (Sisson et al. 1974) in rapid eye movement has been noted. Kron and colleagues (1976) have reported an uncoordinated and ineffective sucking reflex as a manifestation of the opioid abstinence syndrome, whereas Lodge and colleagues (1975) found that the withdrawal period was characterized by heightened auditory responsiveness and orientation, lowered overall alertness, and poor attentiveness to visual stimuli.

Differences in neurological status between opioid-dependent and control groups have not been noted by some workers (Kaltenback et al. 1979). However, Rosen and Johnson (1982a) reported tone discrepancies, developmental delays, and eye problems in children up to 18 months of age delivered by methadone-dependent mothers. Between 6 and 12 months, no real language development was detected.

Beyond the withdrawal period, Wilson et al. (1973) have found adaptive behavior, language performance, and personal-social development of heroin-exposed children to be normal, but gross motor coordination was more advanced than fine motor coordination. Disturbances of activity levels and/or attention span, along with sleep disturbances, temper tantrums, and low tolerance to frustration were recorded by Wilson at 1 year, while the onset of hyperactivity began at 12 to 18 months. Using the Bayley Scale of Infant Behavior as a monitor for mental and motor development, a number of investigators have found children that subjected perinatally to opioids are within the normal range (Blatman and Lipsitz 1972; Chasnoff et al. 1980). However, Wilson et al. (1981) have noted the less attentive nature of both methadone- and heroin-exposed infants, while Kaltenbach et al. (1979) recorded a higher failure rate on three specific items: naming of two objects, pointing to five pictures, and naming of three objects. Kaltenbach suggested that subtle differences in cognitive behavior occur in opioid-exposed children that may be occluded by summary scores. Rosen and Johnson (1982a) reported a lower than normal score for methadone-exposed infants on both the mental and motor development indices at 12 and 18 months of age, and Strauss et al. (1976) also noted delays in the physical development index.

Opioid-subjected infants tested on the Gesell scales (Finnegan et al. 1977; Wilson et al. 1973), Merrill-Palmer test, and Peabody Picture Vocabulary test (Blatman and Lipsitz 1972), as well as the Object Permanence Scales (Rosen and Johnson 1982), appeared normal. A number of workers have reported disorders in speech and/or language development (Blatman and Lipsitz 1972) in children subjected to opioids, although Lodge et al. (1975) reported strength in the realm of language for methadone-exposed offspring.

Few studies that extend beyond the first few years of childhood have been conducted on children maternally subjected to opioids. Nichtern (1973), examining children up to 15 years of age born of heroin-dependent mothers, recorded a number of problems related to their capacity for human relationships, demonstration of excessive adult-peer interactions, poor socialization, and the use of withdrawal to deal with difficult situations. Rosen and Johnson (1982a), in a study of children exposed in utero to methadone, recorded signs of impaired development, including smaller head circumferences, strabismus and/or nystagmus, and abnormalities in muscle tone, coordination, and language. Strauss et al. (1979) found a cluster of behavioral differences related to greater task-irrelevant activity in methadone-exposed children during testing situations. These authors suggest that in structured and demanding situations, qualities of attentiveness and motor inhibition may be a domain in which opioid-exposed children might reveal particular vulnerabilities.

The neurobehavioral implications of exposure to heroin during early life have been reported by Wilson and colleagues (1979). Wilson did not find problems with speech and language function, but on a battery of perceptual measures, visual, tactile, and auditory perception were less than normal. Moreover, the parents of these children noted difficulties for their heroin-exposed children in the areas of self adjustment, social adjustment, and physical adjustment. Items included were: uncontrolled temper, impulsiveness, poor self-confidence, aggressiveness, and difficulty in making and keeping friends. These children were very active, although ratings of attention, cooperation, and alertness were not abnormal. Wilson concludes that heroin-exposed children may have a problem common to the general process of perception rather than a specific sensory deficit, and feels that behavioral problems in these children may be manifestations of "impaired attention and organizational abilities."

In addition to the neurobehavioral sequelae described for children born of opioid-dependent women, a number of studies have monitored growth. Some studies (Blatman and Lipsitz 1972) reveal no abnormalities, while others (Strauss et al. 1976; Wilson et al. 1981; Finnegan 1981) have recorded lower (but not significantly reliable) values for offspring exposed to opioids. A substantial number of reports (Wilson et al. 1973; Wilson 1975; Ting et al. 1974, 1978; Rosen and Johnson 1982a, 1982b; Chasnoff et al. 1982) document delayed growth properties associated with perinatal opioid exposure. These delays may take the form of noticeably lower body weights, shorter body lengths (height), and/or smaller head circumferences.

As in most areas of human research, data collection and interpretation are often fraught with difficulties. In the study of perinatal opioid exposure and human development, the potential for problems is further compounded. The licit and illicit use of opioids so alters psychological, behavioral, and physiological processes that it elevates the drug to a paramount position in the life of any user. These individuals consume opioids during pregnancy despite the ramifications of such consumption on the health of their children. Moreover, the study of opioid exposure in developing humans really involves two individuals: mother and offspring; in some cases, other individuals (e.g., caregivers) may also be involved. Thus, the interaction of these forces only serves to potentially confuse essential issues further. Fortunately, in the case of clinical studies on opioids and development, recognition of and discussion about problems in experimental design and interpretation have not been overlooked (e.g., Householder et al. 1982; Strauss et al. 1979; Wilson et al. 1981; Aylward 1982). Some of these confounding variables include: polydrug abuse, poor prenatal and/or postnatal care, demographics, socioeconomic states, length of hospitalization, neonatal withdrawal, breast feeding, mother-infant/child interpretations, paternal influences, sample selection, type of tests used for investigation, structuring of appropriate comparison groups, "dropout" rate of patients in the study, and statistical analysis.

Rather than being overwhelmed by these confounding variables and simply dismissing reports cited in this review, one needs to be aware that although the goal of clinical research may be to determine a relationship between cause and effects, this type of distinction may be unattainable. Searching for the etiology of opioid-related problems (much less defining all specific abnormalities) could be unrewarding. Given all of the possible confounding variables enumerated above, it is therefore no wonder that defining pathognomonic features of perinatal opioid exposure is a very difficult task. A fine example of the problems in attempting to ascribe specific characteristics to perinatal opioid exposure concerns the neonatal abstinence syndrome. Neonatal withdrawal has been considered to be a hallmark sign of maternal opioid consumption; yet, a variety of nonopioid drugs consumed by the mother can elicit somewhat similar effects. Some of these agents include alcohol, barbiturates, chlordiazepoxide, clomipramine, ethchlorvynol, glutethimide, hydroxyzine, and meprobamate (Committee on Drugs 1983). Thus, at least in the clinical realm, we may have to be satisfied with the knowledge that opioids are part of a cumulative effect from an overall potentially dangerous milieu that contributes to any damaging sequelae encountered.

Laboratory Observations

Laboratory studies offer another perspective as to the influences of opioids on development. Through laboratory investigations, the goal of achieving information in regard to opioids and biological development can be realized. Laboratory models also allow us to address these questions in a wide variety of methodologies that include, in addition to maternal models of opioid consumption, studies in postnatally developing animals, regenerating tissues, tissues and cells in culture, and in other in vitro preparations. Thus, the laboratory has allowed workers to be unrestricted in their designs, yet to be able to cast light on the essential biological question being asked: Do opioids influence development and, if so, how?

Just as in the earlier synopsis of the clinical literature, it simply is beyond the scope of this paper to review all of the laboratory literature. Once again, the reader should be aware of a series of bibliographies (Zagon et al. 1982, 1984) that can serve as a guide to any laboratory (and clinical) topic desired. Moreover, the reader can consult a recent review of the neurobehavioral sequelae associated with perinatal opioid exposure by Zagon and McLaughlin (1984a). In the following discussion, some of the highlights of the laboratory literature will be mentioned.

In regard to studies that have attempted to create a "model" of maternal opioid consumption to determine the effects on offspring, it should be clearly recognized that a variety of routes of administration, drug dosages, and schedules of treatment have been employed. Maternal exposure to opioids does appear to have little effect on estrous cycle, fertility, length of gestation, and parturition (e.g., Zagon and McLaughlin 1977a, 1977b, 1977c), although difficulties with conception and a protraction of the gestational period (Buchenauer et al. 1974), as well as positional malformations of the fetus (Chandler et al. 1975) have been recorded. A distinct effect of maternal opioid consumption appears to be a reduction in maternal body weight during pregnancy (McGinty and Ford 1976; White et al. 1978; Seidler et al. 1982; Zagon and McLaughlin 1977a), but these weight deficits do not appear to be caused by insufficient nutritional status (Ford and Rhines 1979; White et al. 1978). In general, maternal exposure to morphine and methadone (Davis and Lin 1972; Zagon and McLaughlin 1977b, 1977d) does not have a detrimental influence on litter size, although some decreases in litter size with higher doses of methadone have been noted (Middaugh and Simpson 1980). Teratogenicity appears to be associated with high drug dosages administered acutely or over a short time period (Geber and Schramm 1975), but not with lower dosages administered chronically. Some increase in stillborns has been observed with high drug dosages (Freeman 1980; Sobrian 1977), while other studies reveal little problem in this area (Davis and Lin 1972).

The effect of transplacental exposure to opioids on infant viability is determined by drug dosage and whether or not the neonates continue to receive opioids postnatally (e.g., breast milk, direct injection). Neonates that do not continue to receive opioids often may be hypersensitive to stimuli and experience tremors at birth, with notable infant mortality found in the first few days of life for those pups exposed to morphine, heroin, methadone, and levo-alpha-acetylmethadol (LAAM) (e.g., Davis and Lin 1972; Zagon and McLaughlin 1977d; Freeman 1980).

Since the timetable of behavioral maturation in rodents is so well known, evaluation of the developmental pattern in opioid-exposed offspring can be determined (Zagon and McLaughlin 1978b). Delays in physical characteristics (e.g., eye opening), spontaneous motor physical characteristics (e.g., walking), and reflexive tests (e.g., visual orientation) have all been noted. Interestingly, animals exposed only prenatally to opioids (i.e., allowed to go through withdrawal at birth and not receiving drug postnatally) exhibit the greatest number of delays in attaining behavioral capacities and physical characteristics. Those animals receiving drug prenatally and postnatally (a situation somewhat comparable to that in humans when therapeutic intervention prevents withdrawal) are often closest to the normal timetable of maturation.

In the rat, behavior in the period shortly after weaning (postnatal days 21 to 44) has generally been characterized by a reduction in activity and a decreased emotionality relative to control offspring (Freeman 1980; Grove et al. 1979; Zagon et al. 1979a). Zagon and McLaughlin (1981b) have also found an abnormally high incidence of wet-dog-shake and head-shake behaviors during this period that resembled drug withdrawal. In contrast to the reduced activity levels in opioid-treated pups at weaning, young adults (postnatal days 45 to 89) generally were hyperactive and more emotional (Davis and Lin 1972; Grove et al. 1979; Zagon et al. 1979a). Once again, methadone-exposed pups often exhibited head-shake and wet-dog-shake behaviors, suggesting a protracted phase of withdrawal. Peters (1978) has also accumulated preliminary evidence of learning disabilities in methadone- and morphine-exposed rats at this age.

Adult rats that were perinatally exposed to opioids exhibit a lasting impairment in the ability to acquire fear (Sonderegger and Zimmerman 1976), a reduction in social dominance (Thompson and Zagon 1982), problems in learning (Middaugh and Simpson 1980; Zagon et al. 1979b), and a facilitation toward self-administrative behavior (Rech et al. 1980).

In regard to other anatomical, physiological, and biochemical correlates to opioid exposure in early life, a number of important observations have been made. Somatic growth retardation (e.g., McLaughlin and Zagon 1980; McLaughlin et al. 1978; Slotkin et al. 1976, 1980), smaller brain dimensions (Zagon and McLaughlin 1977b, 1978a), and deficits in organ weights (McLaughlin and Zagon 1980; McLaughlin et al. 1978) have been reported. Physiological dysfunction in regard to thermoregulation (Thompson and Zagon 1981; Thompson et al. 1979), nociceptive thresholds (Zagon and McLaughlin 1980, 1981a, 1982b), and aberrant response to opioids and nonopioid drugs (Zagon and McLaughlin 1981a, 1984b) have also been recorded. Opioid-exposed offspring, particularly those subjected to drugs only prenatally, often exhibit deficits in brain cell number, as well as alterations in brain RNA and protein concentrations and content (Zagon and McLaughlin 1978a). Changes in polyamine metabolism (Slotkin et al. 1976, 1979) and in the ontogeny of catecholaminergic systems, as well as a retardation in the synaptic development of 5-hydroxytryptamine, dopamine, and epinephrine neurons in the nervous system have been cited (McGinty and Ford 1980; Rech et al. 1980; Slotkin et al. 1982). Morphological investigations have shown that the timetable of neurogenesis is dependent on the schedule of drug exposure (Zagon and McLaughlin 1982b), and that prenatal exposure to opioids is related to reductions in cortical thickness and number of cells in the neocortex during the first 2 weeks of rat development, in addition to neuronal density changes in the hippocampus up to postnatal day 28 (Ford and Rhines 1979). It does not appear that either maternal undernutrition or inadequate nutrition of the offspring form the etiologic basis for opioid-related problems (e.g., Ford and Rhines 1979; Zagon and McLaughlin 1982a; McLaughlin and Zagon 1980; Seidler et al. 1982; White et al. 1978; Raye et al. 1977; Smith et al. 1977). Moreover, hypoxia due to opioid consumption does not appear to be responsible for the sequelae recorded (White and Zagon 1979).

Comparisons of Clinical and Laboratory Findings

Information discussed in this review and others (Zagon and McLaughlin 1983a, 1983b, 1983c, 1983d, 1984a), as well as inspection of individual papers on the subject (see Zagon et al. 1982, 1984), reveals a number of striking parallels between clinical and laboratory findings. In summary fashion, these include: passive dependence of the fetus on opioids, occurrence of the neonatal abstinence syndrome, high rate of morbidity and mortality of the neonate when not given supportive therapy for withdrawal, sleep disturbances in the neonate, protracted/subacute withdrawal, delays in sensorimotor development, retardation in somatic growth, smaller head circumferences in humans/smaller brain sizes in laboratory animals, delays in walking, problems in visual and/or auditory systems, abnormalities in neuropathological studies indicating alterations in neuro-ontogeny, diminished alertness, poor attention spans in early phases of development, hyperactivity in later phases of development, learning disabilities, and social maladjustments.

Etiological Considerations of the Perinatal Opioid Syndrome

Although many studies to date have dealt more with the phenomenological aspects of opioids and development, they all have, to some degree or another, helped formulate a picture contributing to the uncovering of the etiology and pathogenesis associated with the perinatal opioid syndrome. Information garnered from other biological studies on opioids and early life also should be mentioned before attempting to place this syndrome in perspective. First, opioids are known to selectively accumulate in the brains and nervous tissues of fetal rats (Peters et al. 1972) and preweaning rats (Shah and Donald 1979), presumably because developing organisms have an increased permeability of the blood-brain barrier. Moreover, opioids have been reported to exert a stereospecific effect on growth in animals (Smith et al. 1977; Crofford and Smith 1973), indicating that opioid action is quite specific. The effects of opioids also have been shown to be blocked by concomitant administration of opioid antagonists such as naloxone (Crofford and Smith), suggesting that opioid action resides at the level of the opiate receptor. In this regard, it should be noted that opiate receptors have been found in body and brain tissues of developing organisms (e.g., Gibson and Vernadakis 1982; Clendeninn et al. 1976).

Tissue culture studies in our laboratory (Zagon and McLaughlin 1984c; McLaughlin and Zagon 1984) have verified stereospecific and naloxone-reversible effects of opioid agonists on cell growth, and also reveal that tolerance can develop to these influences. Additionally, cells that are physically dependent on opioid agonists and withdrawn from drugs go through a withdrawal. A principle manifestation of cellular withdrawal is a diminution in mitotic activity.

Thus, it could be conjectured that opioid agonists serve to inhibit growth at the locus of the opioid receptor. The relationship of the receptor to growth remains an exciting new frontier for exploration. In the case of maternal opioid agonist consumption, it can be envisioned that these agonists depress developmental events until the cells are able to become tolerant to drug exposure. The magnitude of prenatal effects on growth depends on the drug dosage and the length of time needed to establish tolerance in the developing organism. Withdrawal from opioid agonist exposure at birth (or even during fetal life) would force developing cells to readjust to an absence of drug, which would result in a delayed growth profile; the extent of these delays would correlate with the magnitude of withdrawal. Amelioration of withdrawal at birth by administration (breast feeding or direct administration) of opioid agonistlike agents would circumvent the need for readjustment and allow the cells and tissue to continue developing in an established (albeit, containing opioid agonist) milieu. This hypothesis fits very nicely with laboratory findings that prenatal exposure followed by postnatal withdrawal is most detrimental to development, whereas prenatal exposure along with administration of opioids in the postnatal life usually exerts the least short- and long-term damage. In the clinical setting, elimination or at least minimization of the withdrawal syndrome probably attenuates many detrimental influences. Therefore, it is hardly any wonder that difficulties might exist in establishing firm evidence separating the effects of perinatal opioid exposure from other potentially damaging influences.

NEW LESSONS

If indeed exogenous opioids such as methadone, heroin, and morphine can inhibit growth by acting stereospecifically and in a naloxone-reversible fashion at the level of the opiate receptor, then the question arises as to whether the body's own morphine--the endorphins--could also regulate growth by interaction with opiate receptors known to be present on developing cells. To investigate this possibility further, we administered naltrexone--a potent opioid antagonist--to preweaning rats. Preweaning development in the rat (birth to day 21) is characterized by explosive body and brain growth, and serves as a good model to examine the influences of various agents on developmental events. Daily injections of a relatively high dosage of naltrexone (50 mg/kg) stimulated development in pre-weaning rats, while daily injections of a low dosage (1 mg/kg) inhibited growth (Zagon and McLaughlin 1983a, 1983b, 1984d, 1984e). For example, the body weight of 21-day-old 50 mg/kg naltrexone-treated rats was 18% more than controls and the body weights of 1 mg/kg naltrexone-treated rats was 11% less than controls. Not only were body weights affected, but examination of the wet weights of brain, heart, kidneys, liver, and skeletal muscle were 11 to 32% more than controls for rats in the 50 mg/kg group, and 5 to 24% below normal for animals given 1 mg/kg naltrexone (Zagon and McLaughlin 1983b).

The timing of the appearance of certain physical characteristics that were examined (hair covering, incisor eruption, ear opening, and eye opening) often revealed that many of these traits occurred significantly <u>earlier</u> in the 50 mg/kg naltrexone group, and markedly <u>later</u> in rats receiving 1 mg/kg naltrexone (Zagon and McLaughlin 1983b, 1985). The appearance of spontaneous motor and sensorimotor behaviors was also altered in a similar manner. For example, the initial appearance of walking, a milestone in behavioral ontogeny, appeared 2 days earlier in the 50 mg/kg naltrexone group relative to controls. Furthermore, at the age when only 50% of the controls were able to walk, <u>no</u> rat in the 1 mg/kg naltrexone group could walk, and <u>all</u> (100%) of the animals in the 50 mg/kg naltrexone group could walk (Zagon and McLaughlin 1983b, 1985).

Macroscopic dimensions of the brains and the cerebellum at 21 days of age showed marked increases for the 50 mg/kg naltrexone group and decreases for the 1 mg/kg naltrexone group (Zagon and McLaughlin 1983a, 1984e). Morphometric analysis of the cerebrum revealed a somatosensory cortex in the 50 mg/kg naltrexone group that was 12% thicker than in controls, but 9% thinner in rats of the 1 mg/kg group. In regard to the cerebellum of 21-day-old rats, the 50 mg/kg group had areal measurements of total, molecular layer, internal granule layer, and medullary layer that were 27%, 24%, 28%, and 41%, respectively, greater than controls; animals in the 1 mg/kg group had measurements that were 27%, 30%, 24%, and 27%, respectively, less than those of the control group. The number of neural cells in the molecular layer of rats in the 50 mg/kg group was 76% greater than control levels, and the number of glial cells in the medullary layer was 62% greater in these animals than in control rat cerebella.

Dose-response experiments (Zagon and McLaughlin 1984d) have shown that dosages from 0.1 to 10 mg/kg naltrexone inhibit body and brain growth, whereas dosages of 20 to 100 mg/kg stimulate development. Utilizing opiate challenge experiments (nociceptive response is recorded 30 minutes following an injection of 0.2 mg/kg morphine) to examine the pharmacological efficacy of various daily dosages of naltrexone, dosages of 20 mg/kg or greater were found to block the opioid receptor from interaction with a dose of morphine for 24 hr/day, and dosages of 10 mg/kg naltrexone and less blocked the opioid receptor for only 12 hr/day or less. To further investigate whether the relationship between growth processes, drug dosage, and the pharmacological properties of naltrexone were more than coincidental, some preweaning pups received low dosages (3 mg/kg) of naltrexone given three times daily, which in effect blocked the opiate receptor for 24 hr/day. These rats demonstrated notable increases in body and brain development. A cumulative dosage of 9 mg/kg naltrexone once daily, which blocked the opioid receptor for less than 12 hr/day, retarded growth. Thus, developmental events appear to be governed by the duration of opioid receptor blockade.

These findings, taken together with evidence that endorphins are present in the plasma and brain of developing organisms (Kromer and Teschemacher 1978; Bayon et al. 1979), that immunoreactive analogs of endorphins have been detected in fetal and neonatal cells (Knodel and Richelson 1980; Neale et al. 1978), and that opioid receptors have been identified in brain and body tissues during ontogeny (Coyle and Pert 1976; Gibson and Vernadakis 1982), led us to the exciting and novel proposition that endogenous opioids and their opioid receptors regulate developmental events. These effects on growth do not appear to be due to nutritional or hormonal events (Zagon and McLaughlin 1984d). In fact, we are not aware of any agent (e.g., drug or hormone) or condition that makes a postnatally developing animal larger than "normal" and increases brain development such as we have demonstrated.

The specific mechanisms as to how endogenous opioid systems control growth are unclear. Our studies do show that complete prevention of the interaction between endorphins and opioid receptors by administration of relatively high dosages of naltrexone once daily, or low dosages of naltrexone given repeatedly each day, allows growth to proceed in an "unrestricted fashion" that results in the larger animals. Thus, just as with exogenous opioids such as heroin and methadone, endogenous opioids serve to inhibit growth. Enhancement of this interaction, such as that recorded with temporary opioid receptor blockade by naltrexone administration, results in smaller animals. Although the precise pathways for this diminution in growth are unknown, naltrexone administration has been reported to elevate plasma beta-endorphin levels (Recant et al. 1980) and to increase opioid receptor number and supersensitivity to opioids (Lahti and Collins 1978; Schulz et al. 1979; Tang and Collins 1978; Zukin et al. 1982). In distinction to a total blockade of this interaction, a temporary blockade provides an interval each day when the inhibitory action of basal or elevated levels of endorphins can act on cells possessing a greater complement of opioid receptors. Fascinatingly, naltrexone's effects on infant rat development and the establishment of endogenous opioid control of growth is consistent with other studies in which endogenous opioid systems have been demonstrated to control tumorigenesis (Zagon and McLaughlin 1981c, 1981d, 1983c, 1983d, 1984f).

FOOTNOTE

[1]The term opioid is used in the generic sense and refers to exogenous and endogenous substrates, natural or synthetic in origin, that possess opium- or morphine-like properties.

REFERENCES

Abrams, C.A.L. Cytogenetic risks to the offspring of pregnant addicts. Addict Dis 2:63-77, 1975.

Aylward, G.P. Methadone outcome studies: Is it more than the methadone? J Pediatr 101:214-215, 1982.

Bayon, A.; Shoemaker, W.J.; Bloom, F.E.; Mauss, A.; and Guillemin, R. Perinatal development of the endorphin and enkephalin-containing systems in the rat brain. Brain Res 179:93-101, 1979.

Blatman, S., and Lipsitz, P.J. Children of women maintained on methadone: accidental methadone poisoning of children. In: Proceedings of the Fourth National Conference on Methadone Treatment. New York: NAPAN. 1972. pp. 175-176.

Blinick, G.; Inturrisi, C.E.; Jerez, E.; and Wallach, R.C. Methadone assays in pregnant women and progeny. Am J Obstet Gynecol 121:617-621, 1975.

Blum, R.H. A history of opium. In: Blum, R.H. and Associates, Society and Drugs. I. Social and Cultural Observations. San Francisco: Jossey-Bass Inc., 1969. pp. 45-58.

Buchenauer, C.; Turnbow, M.; and Peters, M.A. Effect of chronic methadone administration on pregnant rats and their offspring. J Pharmacol Exp Ther 189:66-71, 1974.

Bureau, A. Accouchement d'une morphinomane: prevue chimique du passage de la morphine a travers le placenta: reflexions. Bull Mem Soc Obstete Gynecol 356-362, 1895.

Carr, J.N. Drug patterns among drug-addicted mothers: incidence, variance in use, and effects on children. Pediatr Ann 4:408-417, 1975.

Chandler, J.M.; Robie, P.; Schoolar, J.; and Desmond, M.M. The effects of methadone on maternal-fetal interactions in the rat. J Pharmacol Exp Ther 192:549-554, 1975.

Chasnoff, I.J.; Hatcher, R.; and Burns, W.J. Early growth patterns of methadone-addicted infants. Am J Dis Child 134:1049-1051, 1980.

Chasnoff, I.J.; Hatcher, R.; and Burns, W.J. Polydrug- and methadone-addicted newborns: a continuum of impairment? Pediatrics 70:210-213, 1982.

Chavez, C.J.; Ostrea, E.M.; Stryker, J.C.; and Smialek, A. Sudden infant death syndrome among infants of drug-dependent mothers. J Pediatr 95:407-409, 1979.

Clendeninn, N.J.; Petraitis, M.; and Simon, E. J. Ontological development of opiate receptors in rodent brain. Brain Res 118:157-160, 1976.

Committee on Drugs. Neonatal drug withdrawal. Pediatrics 72:895-902, 1983.

Coyle, J.T. , and Pert, C.B. Ontogenetic development of [^{3}H]naloxone binding in rat brain Neuropharmacology 15:555-560, 1976.

Crofford, M., and Smith, A.A. Growth retardation in young mice treated with dl-methadone. Science 181:947-949, 1973.

Davis, W.M., and Lin, C.H. Prenatal morphine effects on survival and behavior of rat offspring. Res Commun Chem Pathol Pharmacol 3:205-214, 1972.

Davis, W.M., and Shanks, B. Neurological aspects of perinatal narcotic addiction and methadone treatment. Addict Dis 2:213-226, 1975.

Desmond, M.M., and Wilson, G.S. Neonatal abstinence syndrome: Recognition and diagnosis. Addict Dis 2:112-121, 1975.

Dinges, D.F.; Davis, M.M.; and Glass, P. Fetal exposure to narcotics: Neonatal sleep as a measure of nervous system disturbance. Science 209:619-621, 1980.

Dole, V.P., and Nyswander, M.A. Medical treatment for diacetyl-morphine (heroin) addiction. JAMA 193:646-650, 1965.

Earle, F.B. Maternal opium habit and infant mortality. M Standard (Chicago) 3:2, 1888.

Finnegan, L.L. The effects of narcotics and alcohol on pregnancy and the newborn. Ann NY Acad Sci 362:136-157, 1981.

Finnegan, L.P.; Connaughton, J.F.; Emich, J.P.; and Wieland, W. Comprehensive care of the pregnant addict and its effect on maternal and infant outcome. In: Committee on Problems of Drug Dependence (34th Annual Scientific Meeting), Ann Arbor, MI, 1972. pp. 372-390.

Finnegan, L.L.; Reeser, D.S.; Ting, R.Y.; Rozenzwerg, M.; and Keller, A. Growth and development of children born to women maintained on methadone during pregnancy. Pediatr Res 11:377, 1977.

Ford, D., and Rhines, R. Prenatal exposure to methadone HCl in relationship to body and brain growth in the rat. Acta Neurol Scand 59:248-262, 1979.

Freeman, P.R. Methadone exposure in utero: effects on open-field activity in weanling rats. Int J Neurosci 11:295-300, 1980

Geber, W. F., and Schramm, L.C. Congenital malformations of the central nervous system produced by narcotic analgesics in the hamster. Am J Obstet Gynecol 123:705-713, 1975.

Gibson, D.A., and Vernadakis, A. [^{3}H]Etorphine binding activity in early chick embryos: brain and body tissue. Brain Res 4:23-29, 1982.

Glass, L.; Rajegowda, B.K.; and Evans, H.E. Absence of respiratory distress syndrome in premature infants of heroin-addicted mothers. Lancet II:685-686, 1971.

Goodfriend, M.J.; Shey, I.A.; and Klein, M.D. The effects of maternal narcotic addiction on the newborn. Am J Obstet Gynecol 71:29-36, 1956.

Graham-Mulhall, S. Opium the Demon Flower. New York: Harold Vinal (reprinted in 1981 by Arno Press Inc.), 1926.

Grove, L.V.; Etkin, M.K.; and Rosencrans, J.A. Behavioral effects of fetal and neonatal exposure to methadone in the rat. Neurobehav Toxicol 1:87-95, 1979.

Householder, J.; Hatcher, R.; Burns, W.; and Chasnoff, I. Infants born to narcotic-addicted mothers. Psychol Bull 92:453-468, 1982.

Kaltenbach, K.; Graziani, L.T.; and Finnegan, L.P. Methadone exposure in utero: developmental status at one and two years of age. Pharmacol Biochem Behav 11(Supp):15-17, 1979.

Kandall, S.R., and Gartner, L.M. Late presentation of drug withdrawal symptoms in newborns. Am J Dis Child 27:58-61, 1974.

Knodel, E.L., and Richelson, E. Methionine-enkephalin immunoreactivity reactivity in fetal rat brain cells in aggregating culture and in mouse neuroblastoma cells. Brain Res 197:565-570, 1980.

Kromer, W., and Teschemacher, H. An opiate withdrawal-like phenomenon in the fetal guinea pig ileum upon naloxone challenge. Eur J Pharmacol 49:445-446, 1978.

Kron, R.E.; Litt, M.; Phoenix, M.D.; and Finnegan, L.P. Neonatal narcotic narcotic abstinence: effects of pharmacotherapeutic agents and maternal drug usage on nutritive suckling behavior. J Pediatr 88:637-641, 1976.

Laase, C.F.J. Narcotic drug addiction in the newborn, report of a case. Am J Med 25:283-286, 1919.

Lahti, R.A., and Collins, R.J. Chronic naloxone results in prolonged increases in opiate binding sites in brain. Eur J Pharmacol 51:185-186, 1978.

Langstein, L. Uber das schicksal von morphiumsuchtigen frauen geborener sauglinge. Med Klin 26:500-501, 1930.

Lichenstein, P.M. Infant drug addiction. NY Med J 15:905, 1915.

Lodge, A. Developmental findings with infants born to mothers on methadone maintenance: a preliminary report. In: Beschner, G., and Brotman, R., eds. NIDA Symposium on Comprehensive Health Care for Addicted Families and Their Children. DHEW Pub. No. (ADM) 78-480. Washington, D.C.: Supt. of Docs., U.S. Govt. Print. Off., 1977. pp 79-85.

Lodge, A.; Marcus, M.M.; and Ramer, C.M. Neonatal addiction: a two-year study. II. Behavioral and electrophysiological characteristics of the addicted neonate. Addict Dis 2:235-255, 1975.

Marcus, J.; Hans, S.L.; and Jeremy, R.J. Differential motor and state functioning in newborns of women on methadone. Neurobehav Toxicol Teratol 4:459-462, 1982.

Martin, E. L'opium, ses abus, mangeurs et fumerus d'opium morphinomanes. Paris, 1893.

McGinty, J.F., and Ford, D.H. The effects of maternal morphine or methadone intake on the growth reflex development and maze behavior of rat offspring. In: Ford, D.H., and Clouet, D.H., eds. Tissue Responses to Addictive Drugs. New York: Spectrum Publications, 1976. pp. 611-629.

McGinty, J.F., and Ford, D.H. Effects of prenatal methadone on rat brain catecholamines. Dev Neurosci 3:224-234, 1980

McLaughlin, P.J., and Zagon, I.S. Body and organ development of young rats maternally exposed to methadone. Biol Neonate 38:15-196, 1980.

McLaughlin, P.J., and Zagon, I.S. Opioid regulation of neurotumor cell growth in vitro. Soc Neuroscience 10:1111, 1984.

McLaughlin, P.J.; Zagon, I.S.; and White, W.J. Perinatal methadone exposure in rats: effects on body and organ development. Biol Neonate 34:48-54, 1978.

Menninger-Lerchenthal, E. Die morphinkrankheit der neugeboren morphinstinscher mutter. Monatsschr Kinderheilkd 60:182-183, 1934.

Middaugh, L.D., and Simpson, L.W. Prenatal maternal methadone effects on pregnant C57BL/6 mice and their offspring. Neurobehav Toxicol 2:307-313, 1980.

Musto, D.F. The American Disease. New Haven: Yale University Press, 1973.

Naeye, R.L.; Blanc, W.; LeBlanc, W.; and Khatamee, M.A. Fetal complications of maternal heroin addiction: abnormal growth, infections, and episodes of stress. J Pediatr 83:1055-1061, 1973.

Neale, J.H.; Barker, J.L.; Uhl, G.R.; and Snyder, S.H. Enkephalin-containing neurons visualized in spinal cord cell cultures. Science 201:467-469, 1978.

Nichtern, S. The children of drug users. J Am Acad Child Psychiatry 12:24-31, 1973.

Ostrea, E.M., and Chavez, C.J. Perinatal problems (excluding neonatal withdrawal) in maternal drug addiction. A study of 830 cases. J Pediatr 94:292-295, 1979.

Perlmutter, J.F. Drug addiction in pregnant women. Am J Obstet Gynecol 99:569-572, 1967.

Perlmutter, J.F. Heroin addiction and pregnancy. Obstet Gynecol Surv 29:439-446, 1974.

Perlstein, M.A. Congenital morphinism. A rare cause of convulsions in the newborn. JAMA 135:633, 1947.

Peters, M.A. A comparative study on the behavioral response of offspring of female rats chronically treated with methadone and morphine. Proc West Pharmacol Soc 21:411-418, 1978.

Peters, M.A.; Turnbow, M.; and Buchenauer, D. The distribution of methadone in the nonpregnant, pregnant, and fetal rat after acute methadone treatment. J Pharmacol Exp Ther 181:273-278, 1972.

Petty, G.E. Congenital morphinism with report of cases: general treatment of morphinism. Memphis M Monthly 32:37-63, 1912.

Petty, G.E. Narcotic Drug Diseases and Allied Ailments. Tennessee: J.A. Davis, Co., 1913.

Raye, J.R.; Dubin, J.W.; and Blechner, J.N. Fetal growth retardation following maternal morphine administration: nutrition or drug effects? Biol Neonate 32: 222-228, 1977.

Recant, L.; Voyles, N.R.; Luciano, M.; and Pert, C.B. Naltrexone reduces weight gain, alters "ß-endorphin", and reduces insulin output from pancreatic islets of genetically obese mice. Peptides 1:309-313, 1980.

Rech, R.H.; Lomuscio, G.; and Algeri, S. Methadone exposure in utero: effects on brain biogenic amines and behavior. Neurobehav Toxicol 2:75-78, 1980.

Rorke, L.B.; Resser, D.S.; and Finnegan, L.P. Pathological findings in the nervous system of infants born to substance abusing women. In: Problems of Drug Dependence 1977. Cambridge, MA, 1977. pp. 551-571.

Rosen, T.S., and Johnson, H.L. Children of methadone-maintained mothers: follow-up to 18 months of age. J Pediatr 101:192-196, 1982a.

Rosen, T.S., and Johnson, H.L. In utero methadone exposure - three year follow-up. Pediatr Res 16:130A, 1982b.

Sainsbury, H. Drugs and the Drug Habit. London: Methuen Co., 1909.

Salerno, L.J. Prenatal care. In: Rementeria, J.L., ed. Drug Abuse in Pregnancy and Neonatal Effects. St. Louis: C.V. Mosby Co., 1977. pp. 19-29.

Schulman, C.A. Alterations of the sleep cycle in heroin-addicted and "suspect" newborns. Neuropediatrie 1:89-100, 1969.

Schulz, R.; Wuster, M.; and Herz, A. Supersensitivity to opioids following the chronic blockade of endorphin action by naloxone. Naunyn-Schmiedebergs Arch Pharmacol 306:93-96, 1979.

Seidler, F.J.; Whitmore, W.L.; and Slotkin, T.A. Delays in growth and biochemical development of rat brain caused by maternal methadone administration: are the alterations in synaptogenesis and cellular maturation independent of reduced maternal food intake? Dev Neurosci 5:13-18, 1982.

Shah, N.S., and Donald, A.G. Pharmacological effects and metabolic fate of levo-methadone during post-natal development in rat. J Pharmacol Exp Ther 208:491-497, 1979.

Sisson, T.R.C.; Wickler, M.; Tsai, P.; and Rao, I.P. Effects of narcotic withdrawal on neonatal sleep patterns. Pediatr Res 8:451, 1974.

Slotkin, T.A.; Lau, C.; and Bartolome, M. Effects of neonatal or maternal methadone administration on ornithine decarboxylase activity in brain and heart of developing rats. J Pharmacol Exp Ther 199:141-148, 1976.

Slotkin, T.A.; Whitmore, W.L.; Salvaggio, M.; and Seidler, F.J. Perinatal methadone addiction affects brain synaptic development of biogenic amine systems in the rat. Life Sci 24:1223-1230, 1979.

Slotkin, T.A.; Seidler, F.J.; and Whitmore, W.L. Effects of maternal methadone administration on ornithine decarboxylase in brain and heart of the offspring: Relationships of enzyme activity to dose and to growth impairment in the rat. Life Sci 26:861-867, 1980.

Slotkin, T.A.; Weigle, S.J.; Whitmore, W.L.; and Seidler, F.J. Maternal methadone administration: deficient in development of alpha-noradrenergic responses in developing rat brain as assessed by norepinephrine stimulation of ^{33}Pi incorporation into phospholipids in vivo. Biochem Pharmacol 31:1899-1902, 1982.

Smith, A.A.; Hui, F.W.; and Crofford, M.J. Inhibition of growth in young mice treated with d,l-methadone. Eur J Pharmacol 43:307-314, 1977.

Sobrian, S.K. Prenatal morphine administration alters behavioral development in the rat. Pharmacol Biochem Behav 7:285-288, 1977.

Sonderegger, T., and Zimmerman, E. Persistent effects of neonatal addiction in the rat. In: Ford, D.H., and Clouet, D.H., eds. Tissue Responses to Addictive Drugs. New York: Spectrum Publications, 1976. pp. 589-609.

Strauss, M.E.; Andresko, M.; Stryker, J.C.; and Wardell, J.N. Relationship of neonatal withdrawal to maternal methadone dose. Am J Drug Alcohol Abuse 3:339-345, 1976.

Strauss, M.E.; Lessen-Firestone, J.K.; Chavez, C.J.; and Stryker, J.C. Children of methadone-treated women at five years of age. Pharmacol Biochem Behav 11(Supp):3-6, 1979.

Tang, A. H. and Collins, R.J. Enhanced analgesic effects of morphine after chronic administration of naloxone in the rat. Eur J Pharmacol 47:473-474, 1978.

Terry, C.E., and Pellens, M. The Opium Problem. New Jersey: Patterson Smith (originally published in 1928 by the Bureau of Social Hygiene, Inc.), 1970. pp. 312-348.

Thompson, C.I., and Zagon, I.S. Long-term thermoregulatory changes following perinatal methadone exposure in rats. Pharmacol Biochem Behav 14:653-659, 1981.

Thompson, C.I., and Zagon, I.S. Decreased dominance in adult rats perinatally exposed to methadone. Paper presented at the Eastern Psychological Assoc., Baltimore, MD, 1982.

Thompson, C.I.; Zagon, I.S.; and McLaughlin, P.J. Impaired thermal regulation in juvenile rats following perinatal methadone exposure. Pharmacol Biochem Behav 10:551-556, 1979.

Ting, R.; Keller, A.; Berman, P.; and Finnegan, L.P. Follow-up studies of infants born to methadone-dependent mothers. Pediatr Res 8:436, 1974.

Ting, R.Y.; Keller, A.; and Finnegan, L.P. Physical, neurological and developmental assessment of infants born to methadone dependent mothers. In: Schecter, A.; Alksne, H.; Kaufman, E.; Shorty, V.; Henderson, A.; and Lowinson, J.H., eds. Drug Abuse: Modern Trends, Issues, and Perspectives. New York: Marcel Dekker, 1978. pp. 632-641.

White, W.J., and Zagon, I.S. Acute and chronic methadone exposure in adult rats: studies on arterial blood gas concentrations and pH. J Pharmacol Exp Ther 209:451-455, 1979.

White, W.J.; Zagon, I.S.; and McLaughlin, P.J. Effects of chronic methadone treatment on maternal body weight and food and water consumption in rats. Pharmacology 17:227-232, 1978.

Wilson, G.S. Somatic growth effects of perinatal addiction. Addict Dis 2:333-345, 1975.

Wilson, G.S.; Desmond, M.M.; and Verniaud, W.M. Early development of infants of heroin-addicted mothers. Am J Dis Child 126:457-462, 1973.

Wilson, G.S.; McGreary, R.; Kean, J.; and Baxter, J.C. The development of preschool children of heroin-dependent mothers: a controlled study. Pediatrics 63:135-141, 1979.

Wilson, G.S.; Desmond, M.M.; and Wait, R.B. Follow-up of methadone-treated and untreated narcotic-dependent women and their infants: Health, developmental, and social implications. J Pediatr 98:716-722, 1981.

Zagon, I.S. Behavioral effects of prenatal exposure to opiates. In: Schlumpf, M., and Lichstensteiger, W., eds. Drugs and Hormones in Brain Development. Monographs in Neural Sciences 9. Basel: S. Karger, 1983. pp. 159-168.

Zagon, I.S., and McLaughlin, P.J. The effect of chronic maternal methadone exposure on perinatal development. Biol Neonate 31:271-282, 1977a.

Zagon, I.S., and McLaughlin, P.J. The effects of different schedules of methadone treatment on rat brain development. Exp Neurol 56:538-552, 1977b.

Zagon, I.S., and McLaughlin, P.J. The effect of chronic morphine administration on pregnant rats and their offspring. Pharmacology 15:302-310, 1977c.

Zagon, I.S., and McLaughlin, P.J. Morphine and brain growth retardation in the rat. Pharmacology 15:276-282, 1977d.

Zagon, I.S., and McLaughlin, P.J. Perinatal methadone exposure and brain development: A biochemical study. J Neurochem 31:49-54, 1978a.

Zagon, I.S., and McLaughlin, P.J. Perinatal methadone exposure and its influence on the behavioral ontogeny of rats. Pharmacol Biochem Behav 9:665-672, 1978b.

Zagon, I.S., and McLaughlin, P.J. Protracted analgesia in young and adult rats maternally exposed to methadone. Experientia 36:329-330, 1980.

Zagon. I.S., and McLaughlin, P.J. Enhanced sensitivity to methadone in adult rats perinatally exposed to methadone. Life Sci 29:1137-1142, 1981a.

Zagon, I.S., and McLaughlin, P.J. Withdrawal-like symptoms in young and adult rats maternally exposed to methadone. Pharmacol Biochem Behav 15:887-894, 1981b.

Zagon, I.S., and McLaughlin, P.J. Naloxone prolongs survival time of mice treated with neuroblastoma. Life Sci 28:1095-1102, 1981c.

Zagon, I.S., and McLaughlin, P.J. Heroin prolongs survival time and retards tumor growth in mice with neuroblastoma. Brain Res Bull 7:25-32, 1981d.

Zagon, I.S., and McLaughlin, P.J. Comparative effects of postnatal undernutrition and methadone exposure on protein and nucleic acid contents of the brain and cerebellum in rats. Dev Neurosci 5:385-393, 1982a.

Zagon, I.S., and McLaughlin, P.J. Neuronal cell deficits following maternal exposure to methadone in rats. Experientia 38:1214-1216, 1982b.

Zagon, I.S., and McLaughlin, P.J. Analgesia in young and adult rats perinatally exposed to methadone. Neurobehav Toxicol Teratol 4:455-457, 1982c.

Zagon, I.S., and McLaughlin, P.J. Increased brain size and cellular content in infant rats treated with an opiate antagonist. Science 221:1179-1180, 1983a.

Zagon, I.S., and McLaughlin, P.J. Naltrexone modulates growth in infant rats. Life Sci 33:2449-2454, 1983b.

Zagon, I.S., and McLaughlin, P.J. Naltrexone modulates tumor response in mice with neuroblastoma. Science 221:671-673, 1983c.

Zagon, I.S., and McLaughlin, P.J. Opioid antagonists inhibit the growth of metastatic murine neuroblastoma. Cancer Lett 21:89-94, 1983d.

Zagon, I.S., and McLaughlin, P.J. The neurobehavioral sequelae of perinatal opioid addiction: an overview. In: Yanai, J., ed. Neurobehavioral Teratology Amsterdam: Elsevier/North Holland Biomedical Press, 1984a. pp. 197-234.

Zagon, I.S., and McLaughlin, P.J. Prenatal exposure of rats to methadone alters sensitivity to drugs in adulthood. Neurobehav Toxicol Teratol 6:319-324, 1984b.

Zagon, I.S., and McLaughlin, P.J. Opiates alter tumor cell growth and differentiation in vitro. In: Harris, L.S., ed. Problems of Drug Dependence 1983. National Institute on Drug Abuse Research Monograph 49. DHHS Pub. No. (ADM) 84-1316. Washington, D.C.: Supt. of Docs., U.S. Govt. Print Off., 1984c. pp. 344-350.

Zagon, I.S., and McLaughlin, P.J. Naltrexone modulates body and brain development in rats: a role for endogenous opioids in growth. Life Sci 35:2057-2064, 1984d.

Zagon, I.S., and McLaughlin, P.J. Endogenous opioid systems and brain development. In: Caciaglia, F., ed. Physiological and Pharmacological Control of Nervous System Development. Amsterdam: Elsevier/North Holland Biomedical Press, 1984e. pp. 67-70.

Zagon, I.S., and McLaughlin, P.J. Duration of opiate receptor blockade determines tumorigenic responses in mice with neuroblastoma: a role for endogenous opioid systems in cancer. Life Sci 35:409-416, 1984f.

Zagon, I.S., and McLaughlin, P.J. Naltrexone's influence on neurobehavioral development. Pharmacol Biochem Behav, in press (1985).

Zagon, I.S.; McLaughlin, P.J.; and Thompson, C.I. Development of motor activity in young rats following perinatal methadone exposure. Pharmacol Biochem Behav 10:743-749, 1979a.

Zagon, I.S.; McLaughlin, P.J.; and Thompson, C.I. Learning ability in adult female rats perinatally exposed to methadone. Pharmacol Biochem Behav 10:889-894, 1979b.

Zagon, I.S.; McLaughlin, P.J.; Weaver, D.J.; and Zagon, E. Opiates, endorphins, and the developing organism: a comprehensive bibliography. Neurosci Biobehav Rev 6:439-479, 1982.

Zagon, I.S.; McLaughlin, P.J.; and Zagon, E. Opiates, endorphins, and the developing organism: a comprehensive bibliography, 1982-1983. Neurosci Biobehav Rev 8:387-403, 1984.

Zelson, C. Acute management of neonatal addiction. Addict Dis 2:159-168, 1975.

Zelson, C.; Kahn, E.J.; Neumann, L.; and Polk, G. Heroin withdrawal syndrome. J Pediatr 76:483, 1970.

Zelson, C.; Lee, S.T.; and Casalino, M. Neonatal narcotic addiction. N Engl J Med 289:1216-1220, 1973.

Zukin, R.S.; Sugarman, J.R.; Fitz-Syage, M.L.; Gardner, E.L.; Zukin, S.R.; and Gintzler, A.R. Naltrexone-induced opiate receptor supersensitivity. Brain Res 245:285-292, 1982.

ACKNOWLEDGMENTS

The technical and intellectual contributions of P.J. McLaughlin, M.S. to all studies mentioned in this review which originated from our laboratory is gratefully acknowledged. This work was supported in part by grants NS-20500, NS-20623, and NS-21246 from the National Institutes of Health.

AUTHOR

Ian S. Zagon, Ph.D.
Associate Professor of Anatomy
Department of Anatomy
The Milton S. Hershey Medical Center
The Pennsylvania State University
Hershey, PA 17033

Pharmacodynamics of Fetal Exposure to Narcotics

Hazel H. Szeto and Jason G. Umans

INTRODUCTION

Infants born to narcotic addicts are known to be at risk of undergoing an opiate-abstinence syndrome in the neonatal period. The most common manifestations of this syndrome include irritability, hyperactivity, increased eye movements, diarrhea, tachypnea, tremors, exaggerated reflexes, and occasionally generalized seizures. In addition, these infants exhibit abnormal sleep patterns, with an increase in wakefulness and rapid-eye-movement sleep, at the expense of quiet sleep (Glass et al. 1972; Schulman 1969; Dinges et al. 1980).

Although most of the clinical signs of withdrawal subside in a matter of days, some behavioral and neurological disturbances appear to persist into early childhood. Many children have been found to be hyperactive, with shorter attention spans and decreased fine motor coordination (Wilson et al. 1981). These persistent neurological and behavioral effects are often considered consequences of the withdrawal insult. However, it is also possible that prolonged intrauterine exposure to methadone may have direct effects on the development of the nervous system. In both clinical and animal studies, it has been rather difficult to differentiate between direct narcotic effects on fetal development and the consequences of the unavoidable withdrawal syndrome at birth.

Furthermore, it has recently been suggested that the fetus may undergo intermittent intrauterine withdrawal throughout gestation (Lichtblau and Sparber 1981), and this may result in long-term behavioral and neurological disturbances. It is known that detoxification of narcotic addicts during pregnancy results in fetal distress, as evidenced by meconium staining (Hill and Desmond 1963; Harper et al. 1974), increased amniotic fluid catecholamines, and occasional fetal demise (Zuspan et al. 1975). Changes in fetal hemodynamics and meconium staining have also been reported following precipitated morphine withdrawal in pregnant ewes (Cohen et al. 1980). These studies, however, did not examine the behavioral responses which might allow comparison with the abstinence syndrome described in the human neonate. Therefore, although intrauterine opiate withdrawal presents a severe physiologic stress to the fetus, it remains to be determined whether behavioral disturbances are a significant component of the syndrome.

Our objectives were, therefore, to develop an animal model that would permit us to examine the direct effects of morphine exposure in the fetus and to fully characterize the fetal opiate-abstinence syndrome. An understanding of these fundamental pharmacodynamic properties of a narcotic drug in the fetus may provide a better understanding of the long-term effects of narcotics exposure on the developing fetus and neonate.

EXPERIMENTAL METHODS--GENERAL CONSIDERATIONS

The Animal Model

When considering the effects of acute morphine exposure, we are most concerned about its effects on behavioral, respiratory, and cardiovascular functions. This type of information obviously cannot be obtained from the human fetus or the fetus of small laboratory animals. The pregnant sheep, on the other hand, offers a unique opportunity for examining these functional parameters in the fetus under physiologic conditions. The relatively large size of the fetus allows chronic implantation of catheters and electrodes necessary for intrauterine monitoring of behavioral, respiratory, and cardiovascular functions.

The effects of morphine exposure on fetal cardiovascular function can be easily determined with an indwelling catheter in the fetal aorta for continuous monitoring of blood pressure and heart rate.

Respiratory function can be monitored with a pair of electrodes implanted in the diaphragm and a catheter implanted in the trachea. Breathing movements are indicated by a burst of activity in the diaphragmatic electromyogram and a decrease in tracheal pressure.

Effects of drugs on fetal behavioral activity are much more difficult to ascertain since it is not possible to directly observe the fetus. We have recently developed techniques for intrauterine recording of electrocortical activity (ECoG), electromyographic activity (EMG), and eye movements (EOG) in the fetal lamb, making it possible to interpret indirectly from these electrophysiologic measurements the behavioral activity of the fetus (Szeto 1983; Umans and Szeto 1983). Employing the classical criteria for sleep-wake scoring (table 1), we are able to differentiate three distinct states of behavior in the fetal lamb in the third trimester.

TABLE 1

Behavioral State	ECoG	Nuchal EMG	EOG
Arousal	desynchronized	tone, bursts	random, slow
Quiet Sleep	synchronized	tone, bursts	random, slow
Active Sleep	desynchronized	atonia	REMs

Thus, with the development of sophisticated techniques for intrauterine recording of physiologic functions in the fetal lamb, the pregnant sheep has become an ideal animal model for studying both pharmacokinetics and pharmacodynamics of drugs in the maternal-fetal unit. We have previously demonstrated that this model can be used for comparing the extent of fetal exposure to different narcotic drugs (Szeto 1982; Szeto et al. 1978, 1981, 1982).

Experimental Design

In designing any pharmacodynamic study in the fetus, we should ideally have some information regarding the pharmacokinetics of the drug in the maternal-fetal unit. In addition, there are a few points that should be considered in the design of the route and dose of drug administration.

Firstly, since the extent of fetal exposure following maternal drug administration may vary considerably from animal to animal, it is preferable to administer the drug directly to the fetus rather than to the mother. This can be easily accomplished with an indwelling catheter in the fetal vena cava (Szeto et al. 1978). Secondly, if we wish to correlate pharmacodynamic effects with the dose of drug administered, the drug should be administered by constant rate infusion to steady state. This is particularly important when studying periodic events such as sleep-wake behavior (Szeto 1983, Umans and Szeto 1983). Thirdly, a full range of doses should be examined to document dose-related effects and biphasic effects relationships. Single-dose studies may be very misleading, especially if the dose is not within the linear dose range. Finally, for the opiate withdrawal studies, naloxone will be used to precipitate withdrawal in morphine-exposed animals. Naloxone should also be administered directly to the fetus at doses that do not alter any of the measured parameters, and the study should be carried out following different doses of agonist exposure.

EXPERIMENTAL PROCEDURES

Animal Preparation

Thirteen pregnant ewes and their fetuses (gestational ages ranging from 121 to 138 days at the time of study, term being approximately 145 days) were surgically instrumented for monitoring of fetal hemodynamics and behavioral activity at least 5 days prior to study. Details of the surgical procedure have been described previously (Szeto 1983; Umans and Szeto 1983, 1985). Briefly, chronic indwelling catheters were placed in the fetal inferior vena cava for drug infusion and in the distal aorta for continuous monitoring of blood pressure and heart rate. For continuous monitoring of fetal behavioral activity, a pair of stainless steel screws were implanted extradurally over the parietal cortex to record electrocortical activity, a pair of stainless steel screws was implanted over the superior orbital ridge to record eye movements, and stainless steel electrodes were implanted in the dorsal neck muscles and quadriceps femoris muscle to assess nuchal tone and body movements. In addition, fetal breathing movements were monitored via a pair of stainless steel electrodes implanted in the diaphragm and a catheter in the trachea.

Recording Procedures

All recordings of fetal blood pressure (FBP), heart rate (FHR), tracheal pressure (TP), electrocorticogram (ECoG), electromyogram (EMG), and electrooculogram (EOG) were carried out with the ewe standing or lying quietly in an experimental cart with free access to food and water. A companion sheep was kept in the same room to minimize restlessness.

All recordings were obtained with a Gould model 2800 analog recorder and appropriate amplifiers. The ECoG, EMG, and EOG were recorded via Universal amplifiers set at the following filter band widths: ECoG, 0.3 to 30 Hz; EMG, 30 to 300 Hz; and EOG, 1 to 10 Hz.

Drug Protocols

Control recordings of FBP, FHR, and all neurobehavioral parameters were obtained for at least 2 hours prior to drug administration.

In a preliminary study, naloxone was administered intravenously at doses of 0.75, 1.5, 3.0, 6.0, and 12.0 mg to opiate-naive fetuses, without any significant effect on the monitored physiologic variables. We chose a naloxone dose of 6.0 mg for use in all subsequent studies. In previous studies of specific opiate effects, compararable doses precipitated opiate abstinence in rodents (Wei et al. 1973; Umans and Inturrisi 1982).

Morphine was infused to the fetus at a constant rate, ranging from 0.075 to 80.0 mg/hr for 2 to 6 hours. Naloxone was then administered to the fetus at the end of the morphine infusion. All hemodynamic and activity parameters were monitored continuously throughout the control period, during the morphine infusion, and for 2 hours following naloxone administration.

RESULTS

All predrug control recordings showed cyclic variation in electrocortical activity, eye movements, total body movements, and breathing movements (figure 1). Three behavioral states could be clearly distinguished in all recordings according to classic sleep-wake scoring (table 1). During the control period, the fetus spent 85% to 95% of its time alternating between quiet sleep and active sleep. Very short episodes of arousal would sometimes occur during the quiet sleep-active sleep transition or during prolonged periods of quiet sleep.

The administration of morphine to the fetus resulted in two distinct response clusters as a function of dose. At doses lower than 0.30 mg/hr, morphine did not significantly alter any of the measured physiologic parameters. Doses up to 2.5 mg/hr resulted in desynchronization of the ECoG; increased nuchal tone and body and eye movements; continuous fetal breathing movements; and increased heart rate and heart rate variability (figure 2). Higher doses (through 80.0 mg/hr) resulted in a return of synchronized ECoG, accompanied by decreases in body, eye, and breathing movements and heart rate variability (figure 3). These signs of central nervous system depression were evident towards the end of the 2.5 mg/hr infusion in 30% of the animals. Fetal breathing movements were completely suppressed at doses greater than 10 mg/hr. Upon termination of the high-dose infusion, a prolonged period of arousal and enhanced breathing activity was observed before return to control values.

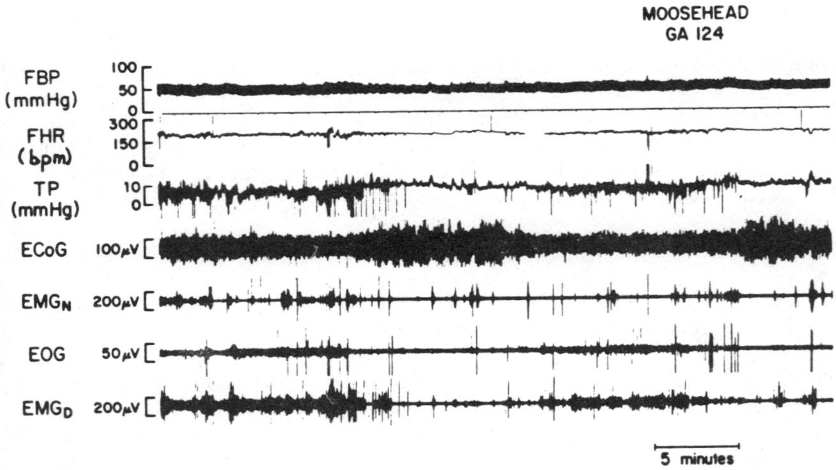

FIGURE 1. Control recording demonstrating cyclic activity in ECoG, Nuchal EMG (EMG_N), EOG, diaphragmatic EMG (EMG_D), and tracheal pressure (TP) prior to morphine exposure.

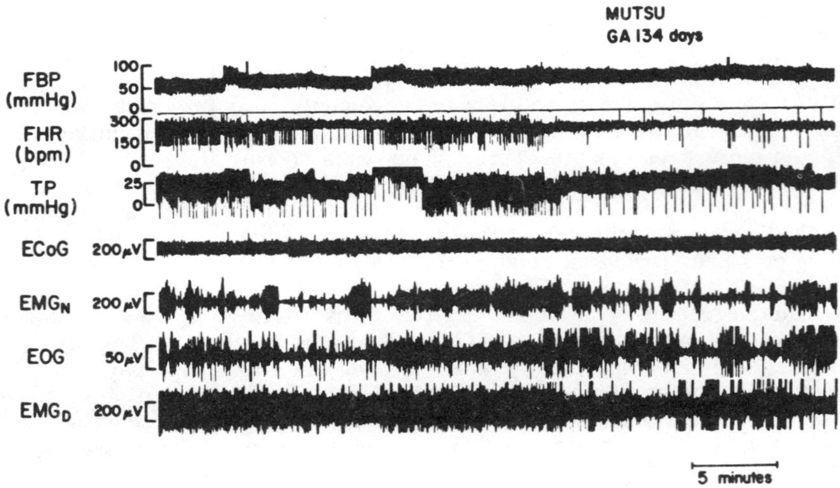

FIGURE 2. Effects of low-dose morphine infusion (2.5 mg/hr) on fetal hemodynamic, behavioral, and respiratory activity. Note continuous fetal arousal and breathing movements.

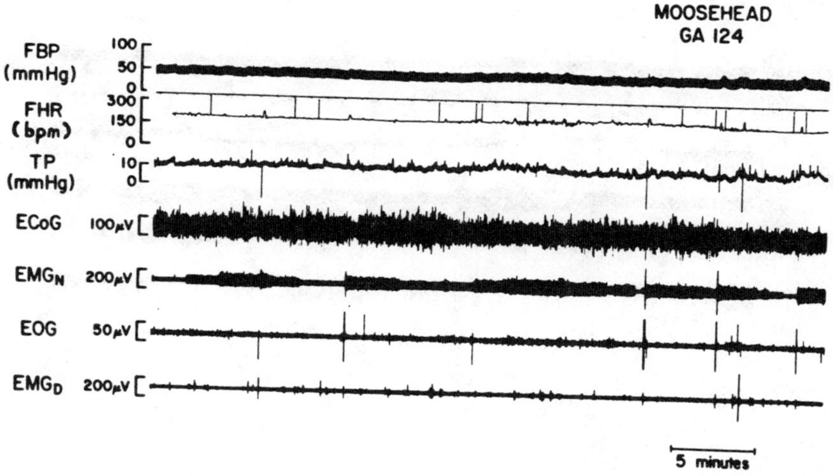

FIGURE 3. Effects of high-dose morphine infusion (25.0 mg/hr) on fetal hemodynamic, behavioral, and respiratory activity. Note prolonged quiet sleep and apnea.

The administration of 6 mg naloxone to opiate-naive fetuses did not result in any alteration in the physiologic parameters which were monitored, or in their pattern of cyclic variation (figure 4).

Following low-dose morphine infusion, naloxone resulted in further desynchronization of the ECoG, an immediate bradycardia, an increase in both the rate and depth of breathing movements, and an increase in total body movements (figure 5). Following high-dose morphine infusion, naloxone provoked a qualitatively similar, but more intense, abstinence syndrome (figure 6).

In fetuses which were subjected to an episode of precipitated abstinence following morphine infusion of 25.0 mg/hr or greater, a second abstinence could be precipitated by naloxone administration 24 hours following the initial withdrawal. Immediately prior to the second dose of naloxone, all fetuses exhibited normal control traces, without evidence of acute opiate effect. The second episode of abstinence was, in each case, similar to, but less intense than, the first.

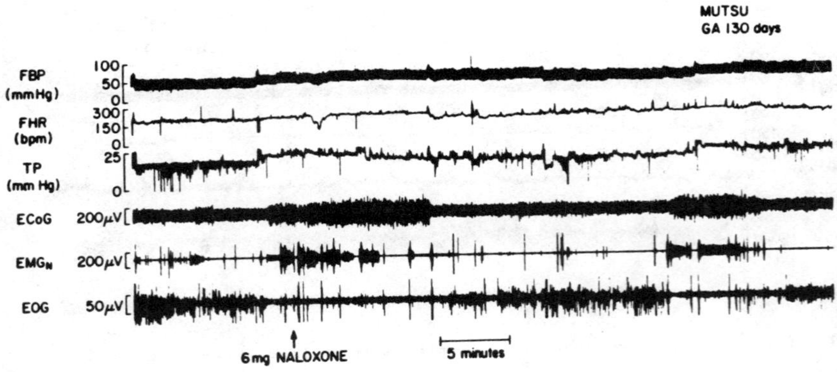

FIGURE 4. The effects of naloxone in an opiate-naive fetus.

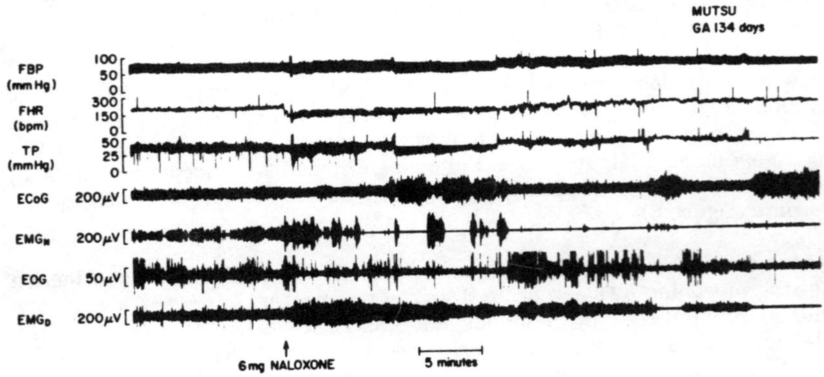

FIGURE 5. The effects of naloxone on fetal hemodynamic and behavioral activity parameters when administered subsequent to a 6-hour infusion of morphine at 2.5 mg/hr.

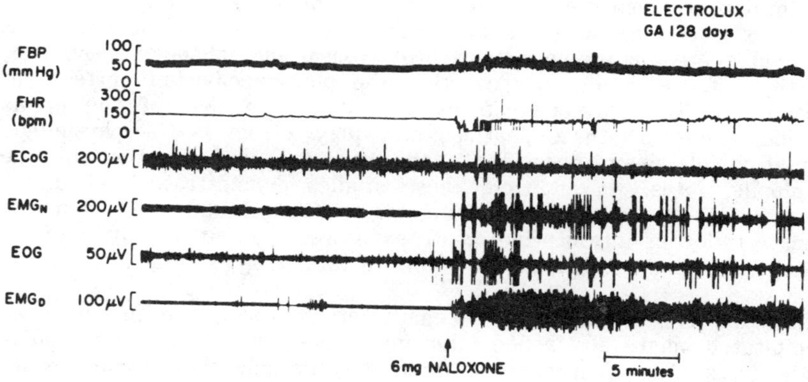

FIGURE 6. The effects of naloxone on fetal hemodynamic and behavioral activity parameters when administered subsequent to a 6-hour infusion of morphine at 25.0 mg/hr.

DISCUSSION

It is generally assumed that neonatal morbidity and developmental abnormalities following intrauterine narcotic exposure result from repeated episodes of fetal withdrawal (Lichtblau and Sparber 1981). Data which suggest that both direct opiate pharmacodynamic effects and fetal withdrawal may contribute significantly to neonatal outcome following intrauterine narcotic exposure is presented below.

Using the chronically instrumented fetal lamb preparation, we have defined the full dose-response relationship of morphine on fetal behavioral, respiratory, and cardiovascular functions. We have previously shown that doses in the range of 2 mg/hr caused complete suppression of quiet sleep in the fetus and induced prolonged episodes of arousal (Umans and Szeto 1983). These arousal periods were associated with continuous breathing movements and increased heart rate and heart rate variability. We have now demonstrated that the morphine dose-response curve is biphasic, with higher doses resulting in quiet sleep and apnea. The biphasic nature of morphine's dose-response curve in the fetus may account for some of the confusion in the current literature, with some investigators reporting a suppression of fetal breathing movements (Rigatto et al. 1984), and others reporting both suppression and stimulation of breathing movements in the fetal lamb (Olsen and Dawes 1984).

We have recently demonstrated a similar biphasic response to a stable enkephalin analog, D-Ala^2-MePhe^4-Met(0)^5-enkephalinol (FK 33-824), in the fetal lamb (Umans et al., in press). At high plasma concentrations, FK 33-824 resulted in apnea and quiet sleep. As plasma concentrations declined, there was prolonged period of arousal and enhanced respiratory activity. These studies suggest that the pharmacodynamic effects of morphine in the developing fetus are similar to that of the opioid peptides, and that these peptides may play a role in the physiologic regulation of sleep, breathing, and cardiovascular function in the developing fetus. In addition, these studies demonstrate that direct effects of opiates may account for some of the effects observed in the neonate following intrauterine opiate exposure, and that the nature of the effect would be dependent on the extent of fetal drug exposure.

In these experiments, we have also characterized a syndrome of naloxone-precipitated opiate abstinence following short-term infusion of morphine to the fetus. The syndrome consists of desynchronization of electrocortical activity; increased total body movements, nuchal tone, and eye movements; continuous rapid, deep breathing movements; an immediate bradycardia associated with transient increases in systolic, diastolic, and pulse pressure; and meconium staining of the amniotic fluid. This syndrome resembles that observed in the human neonate (Glass et al. 1972; Schulman 1969; Dinges et al. 1980). The syndromes differ, however, in that we observed no cortical seizure activity in the fetal lamb. There are no human data available describing the cardiovascular manifestations of neonatal withdrawal.

Based on the present observations, we agree with Zuspan and coworkers (1975) in suggesting that intrauterine opiate withdrawal presents a severe physiologic stress to the developing fetus. Our data, showing that a significant abstinence syndrome may be precipitated following short (2 hours), low-dose fetal exposure to morphine, further suggest that the fetus may undergo a cycle of acute physical dependence and withdrawal following the administration of opiates in normal clinical patients.

In conclusion, we have presented evidence which suggests that both direct opiate pharmacodynamic effects and fetal withdrawal may contribute significantly to neonatal outcome following intrauterine narcotic exposure.

REFERENCES

Cohen, M.S.; Rudolph, A.M.; and Melmon, K.L. Antagonism of morphine by naloxone in pregnant ewes and fetal lambs. Dev Pharmacol Ther 1:58-69, 1980.

Dinges, D.F.; Davis, M.M.; and Glass, P. Fetal exposure to narcotics: neonatal sleep as a measure of nervous system disturbance. Science 209:619-621, 1980.

Glass, L.; Rajegowda, B.K.; and Evans, H.E. Effects of heroin withdrawal on respiratory rate and acid-base status in the newborn. N Engl J Med 186:746-748, 1972.

Harper, R.G.; Solish, G.I.; Purrow, H.M.; Sang, E.; and Panepinto, W.C. The effects of a methadone treatment program upon pregnant heroin addicts and their newborn infants. Pediatrics 54:300-305, 1974.

Hill, R.M., and Desmond, M.M.: Management of the narcotic withdrawal syndrome in the neonate. Pediatr Clin North Am 10:67-86, 1963.

Lichtblau L., and Sparber, S.B. Opiate withdrawal in utero increases neonatal morbidity in the rat. Science 212:943-945, 1981.
Olsen, G.D., and Dawes, G.S. Morphine-induced depression and stimulation of breathing movements in the fetal lamb. In: Jones, C.T., and Nathanielsz, P.W. eds. Physiological Development of Fetus and Newborn. New York: Academic Press, 1984.
Rigatto, H.; Lee, D.; Caces, R.; Albersheim, S; and Moore, M.: The effect of morphine on fetal breathing and behavior. In: Jones, C.T., and Nathanielsz, P.W., eds. Physiological Development of Fetus and Newborn. New York: Academic Press, 1984.
Schulman, C.A. Alterations in the sleep cycle in heroin-addicted and "suspect" newborns. Neuropaediatrie 1:89-100, 1969.
Szeto, H.H. Pharmacokinetics in the ovine maternal-fetal unit. Annu Rev Pharmacol Toxicol 22:221-243, 1982.
Szeto, H.H. Effects of narcotic drugs on fetal behavioral activity: Acute methadone exposure. Am J Obstet Gynecol 146:211-217, 1983.
Szeto, H.H.; Mann, L.I.; Bhakthavathsalan, A.; Liu, M.; and Inturrisi, C.E. Meperidine pharmacokinetics in the maternal-fetal unit. J Pharmacol Exp Ther 206:448-459, 1978.
Szeto, H.H.; Clapp, J.F.; Larrow, R.W.; Hewitt, J.; Inturrisi, C.E.; and Mann, L.I. Disposition of methadone in the ovine maternal-fetal unit. Life Sci 28:2111-2117, 1981.
Szeto, H.H.; Umans, J.G.; and McFarland, J.W. A comparison of morphine and methadone disposition in the maternal-fetal unit. Am J Obstet Gynecol 143:700-706, 1982.
Umans, J.G., and Inturrisi, C.E. Antinociceptive activity and toxicity of meperidine and normeperidine in mice. J Pharmacol Exp Ther 223:203-206, 1982.
Umans, J.G., and Szeto, H.H. Effects of opiates on fetal behavioral activity in utero. Life Sci 33(1):639-642, 1983.
Umans, J.G., and Szeto, H.H. Precipitated opiate abstinence in utero. Am J Obstet Gynecol, 151:441-444, 1985.
Umans, J.G.; Umans, H.R.; and Szeto, H.H. Neurobehavioral activity of a stable enkephalin analogue in the chronically-instrumented fetal lamb. Neurosci Lett, in press.
Wei, E.; Loh, H.H.; and Way, E.L. Quantitative aspects of precipitated abstinence in morphine-dependent rats. J Pharmacol Exp Ther 184:398-403, 1973.
Wilson, G.S.; Desmond, M.M.; and Wait, R.B. Follow-up of methadone- and untreated narcotic-dependent women and their infants: health, developmental and social implications. J Pediatr 98:716-722, 1981.
Zuspan, F.P.; Gumpel, J.A.; Mejia-Zelaya, A.; Madden, J.; and Davis, R. Fetal stress from methadone withdrawal. Am J Obstet Gynecol 122:43-46, 1975.

AUTHORS

Hazel H. Szeto, M.D., Ph.D.
Jason G. Umans, M.D., Ph.D.
Department of Pharmacology
Cornell University Medical College
1300 York Avenue
New York, New York 10021

Positron-Emission Tomography: A New Approach to Feto-Maternal Pharmacokinetics

Bo S. Lindberg, Per Hartvig, Anders Lilja, Hans Lundqvist, Bengt Långström, Petter Malmborg, Anders Rane, Annika Rimland, and Hans Svärd

INTRODUCTION

Positron emission tomography (PET) is a noninvasive technique for studies of the regional kinetics of positron-emitting radiotracers. A drug or other molecule is labeled with short-lived radionuclides such as ^{11}C, ^{13}N, ^{15}O, or ^{18}F. After administration to animal or man, the distribution in the body is visualized by external detectors and the radioactivity concentration in various organs is quantitated as a function of time. With a high specific radioactivity, PET is a true tracer technique and pharmacologic effects of the radiolabeled compound will not occur.

PET has been widely used in studies of brain metabolism where ^{11}C-labeled glucose, glucose analogs, and amino acids are commonly used radiotracers (Ell and Holman 1982). Previously, PET has also been shown to be a valuable tool in studies of tissue distribution of drugs (Hartvig et al. 1984) and studies on receptor-binding kinetics (Wagner et al. 1983).

Studies on the pharmacokinetics and on the metabolism of drugs in the feto-maternal unit in any animal are hampered by the difficulties of obtaining access to the fetal compartments without disturbing the normal function. The close relationship between the placenta and fetal development of humans and some nonhuman primates, such as the rhesus monkey, makes this species an attractive animal model for pharmacokinetic studies during pregnancy. However, the uterus of rhesus monkeys is sensitive to manipulation such as insertion of catheters for fetal blood sampling. In addition, the blood volume of the fetus does not permit withdrawal of more than 5 to 10 ml of blood during an experiment if normal physiologic conditions are to be maintained. A noninvasive technique such as PET would therefore be suitable for the study of rapid transfer of ^{11}C-labeled drugs from the mother to the fetus.

However, PET registers only the distribution of the total radioactivity. If the radiolabeled molecule is metabolized, knowledge of the metabolic pathways is necessary for interpretation of the results. More information can be obtained either by labeling the molecule itself or its metabolites at different sites in different experiments or by the use of additional analytical techniques. Such techniques include chemical and radiochemical analyses (e.g., high performance liquid chromatography [HPLC] and gel chromatography) of blood and other tissue fluids.

The objective of this study was to evaluate the PET technique in combination with other methods in studies of the kinetics of morphine and heroin in pregnant rhesus monkeys. The possibilities and shortcomings of the PET technique in such studies, as well as some preliminary results, are discussed below.

MATERIALS AND METHODS

Radiopharmaceutical Preparation

^{11}C was obtained as [^{11}C]carbon dioxide by using the nuclear reaction $^{14}N(p,\alpha)^{11}C$ and a gas target at the van de Graaff accelerator (11MeV), University of Uppsala. [^{11}C]methyl iodide was prepared as described by Langstrom et al. (1982). The corresponding N-demethylated analogs of morphine and heroin were alkylated and then purified by liquid chromatography. Samples of the purified ^{11}C-labeled compound were analyzed for identity and radiochemical purity by use of reversed-phase liquid chromatography. Radiochemical yields, when corrected for decay, were in the range of 15 to 25%. The time of synthesis, including purification by liquid chromatography, starting with the release of [^{11}C]carbon dioxide was about 50 minutes. Before administration, the samples were filtered through a 0.22 M membrane filter to ensure a sterile preparation. The radioactivity dose was measured immediately before administration. Heroin was used in this experiment with the permission of the Swedish National Board of Health and Welfare.

Animals

Three healthy, well-nourished pregnant rhesus monkeys (Macaca mulatta) from the Primate Laboratory for Reproductive Research in Uppsala were used in the experiments. The age of the animals varied between 7 and 15 years and their weights ranged from 7.3 to 9.1 kg. Gestational age at the time of experiment was 120 to 150 days (pregnancy duration in rhesus monkeys is 167 days). After an overnight fast, the animals were anesthetized with 100 mg ketamine intramuscularly, and the anesthesia was maintained with repeated doses of 50-100 mg ketamine. Two indwelling catheters were placed in different leg veins, one for administration of the drugs and the other for blood sampling. Catheters were also inserted in the bladder and in the amniotic cavity. Ultrasonography was used for visualization of the internal organs of the mother and the fetus . Fetal blood was obtained by ultrasonographic-guided puncture of the umbilical vein (Lindgren and Lindberg, in press). The monkey was fixed in a specially designed cradle and put in the detector opening of the PET in such a way that the radioactivity in the fetal liver and at least one placenta could be simultaneously registered. The experiments were carried out after approval from the Committee for Protection of Laboratory Animals at the University. The animals were not injured by the procedure, the pregnancy continued normally, and the offspring were healthy.

[^{11}C]Morphine (41 μCi and 327 μCi, respectively) and [^{14}C]Morphine (100 μCi; 1.79 μmol; Amersham, England) were simultaneously administered intravenously to two animals. Another monkey was given [^{11}C] heroin (319 μCi) intravenously.

Instrumentation

Imaging of the uterus of the monkey started immediately after administration of the ^{11}C-labeled opiate. A PC 384-3B positron emission tomograph equipped with two rings of detectors (AB Scanditronix, Uppsala, Sweden) was used. Data collection and analyses of images were performed as described by Eriksson et al. (1982). Three horizontal emission images were obtained for 4x10, 4x40, and 200-second periods at predetermined intervals. Each image had a slice thickness of 13 to 14 mm and a spatial resolution of about 8 mm. The resolution of the PET equipment as well as other technical details are given by Bergstrom et al. (1983). The measured radioactivity was corrected for physical decay to the time of administration of the radioactive dose. Uptake--defined as the relative distribution of radioactivity in different organs--was calculated from the corrected radioactivity/cm^3 and divided by the administered radioactivity per gram of body weight where a density of 1 g/cm^3 for all tissues was assumed. A measured uptake of 1.0 indicated that the administered radioactivity was equally distributed in the whole feto-maternal unit.

Sampling and Analysis of Drugs and Metabolites

Maternal blood was collected 0, 5, 15, 30, 60, 90, 120, 180, 240, and 360 minutes after dose. Urine and amniotic fluid were sampled at regular intervals throughout the whole experiment. Fetal blood was obtained from one monkey's umbilical vein at 101 minutes after dose administration.

The ^{11}C activity in the samples was measured immediately in a well counter. The blood samples (about 3 ml) were centrifuged and plasma frozen at -20°C until analyses. [^{14}C]morphine and [^{14}C]Morphine-3-glucuronide ([^{14}C]M3G) were measured by liquid scintillation after collection of fractions using an HPLC method (Svensson et al. 1982). The elimination half-lives were estimated from the concentration-time curve plotted in the log-linear scale.

RESULTS

Positron Emission Tomography

[^{11}C]Morphine was rapidly distributed in the body of the rhesus monkey and maximum uptake was obtained within a few minutes in well-perfused organs, e.g., the placenta (figure 1). The disappearance of the ^{11}C-derived radioactivity in the placenta paralleled the decline of the total ^{11}C-activity in maternal blood. The uptake was slow in the muscles of the mother, as has previously been shown by Hartvig et al. (1984). The [^{11}C]morphine-derived radioactivity was also rapidly transferred to fetal blood and an uptake of 1.5 times equal distribution was seen within 5 to 10 minutes in the fetal liver. The elimination half-life of the ^{11}C-derived radioactivity from the fetal liver was about 20 minutes.

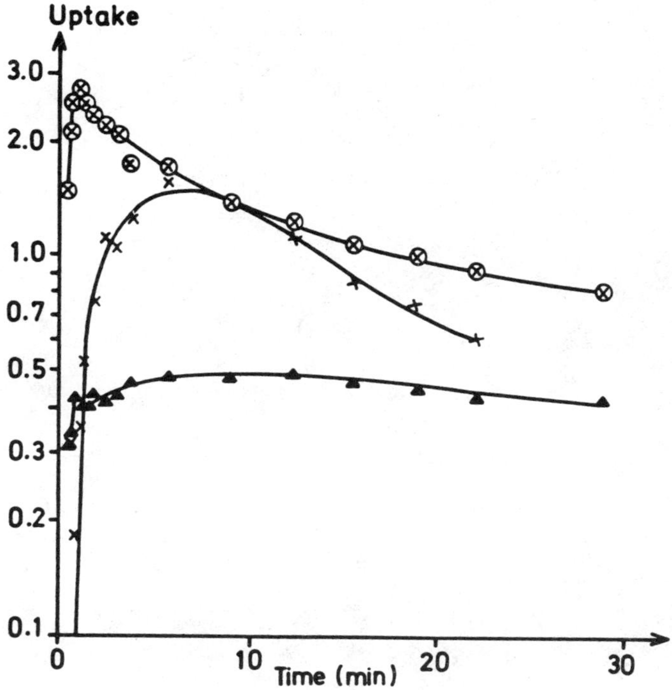

FIGURE 1. Uptake of ^{11}C in placenta and fetal liver after intravenous injection of [^{11}C]morphine to the mother. Uptake is defined as radioactivity per cm^3 tissue in relation to total radioactivity administered per gram body weight. ⊗ denotes the placental uptake; X the fetal liver; and ▲ maternal paraspinal muscle.

Four minutes after administration of [^{11}C]heroin, a maximum radioactivity uptake of 7.5 in the placenta was observed. The uptake of [^{11}C]heroin-derived radioactivity as compared to morphine was even more pronounced in the fetal liver, and an uptake 8 times homogeneous dilution was measured 5 minutes after dose (figure 2). The elimination half-life from the placenta as well as from the fetal liver was estimated to be 15 minutes.

Analysis of Plasma, Urine, and Amniotic Fluid (Figure 3)

[^{14}C]Morphine rapidly left the maternal plasma and was eliminated primarily by conversion to metabolites, e.g., [^{14}C]M3G. Elimination half-lives of [^{14}C]morphine and [^{14}C]M3G in one monkey was 70 and 110 minutes, respectively, whereas in the other monkey, a third very slow elimination phase could be distinguished. The ratios [^{14}C]M3G/[^{14}C] morphine 1 hour after the injection were 8 to 10 in the two mothers. In one experiment, the fetal plasma concentration could be measured 101 minutes after dose. At that moment, the [^{14}C]morphine concentration was 29 μM, or about twice that in maternal plasma (15 μM). The ratio [^{14}C]M3G/[^{14}C]morphine was 5.5 at this time.

483-942 O - 85 - 4 : QL 3

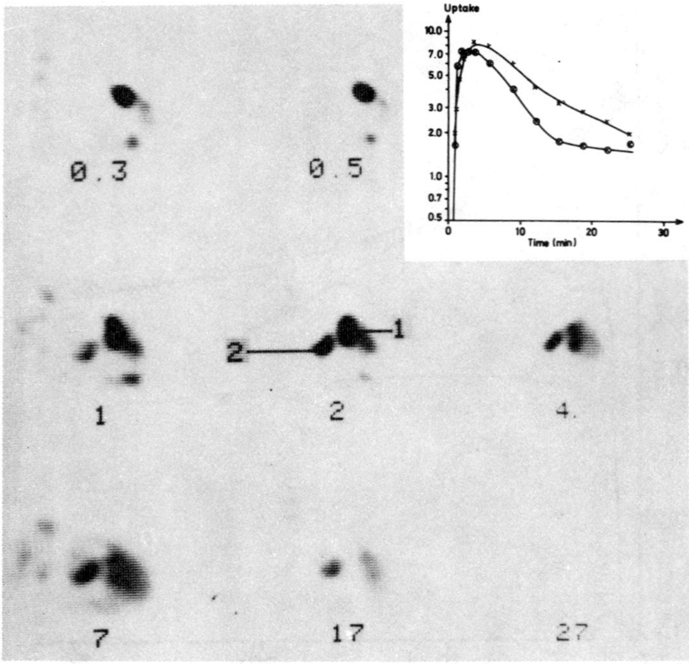

FIGURE 2. PET-images of the distribution of ^{11}C in placenta (1) and fetal liver (2) 0.3–27 min after intravenous administration of [^{11}C]heroin to the mother. To the upper right is shown the uptake in the fetal liver (upper curve), and the placental uptake (lower curve), calculated from regions of interest on the images.

During the 4-hour study period, less than 50% of the administered ^{14}C-derived radioactivity was excreted in the urine, more than 80% of this fraction as [^{14}C]M3G.

Measurable concentrations of [^{14}C]morphine and [^{14}C]M3G from 45 minutes and on indicated the excretion from the fetus into amniotic fluid. [^{14}C]M3G was present at persistently high and constant levels in amniotic fluid for at least the duration of the experiment. In one monkey, a late amniotic fluid sample obtained 16 to 17 hours after dose had the same concentration as at 5 to 6 hours after dose. The ratio between [^{14}C]M3G and [^{14}C]morphine in the amniotic fluid varied between 2 and 3 in both monkeys.

[^{11}C]Morphine-derived radioactivity (^{11}C-activity) was measurable in maternal blood and urine for at least 3 hours (figure 4). The increasing ^{11}C-activity in amniotic fluid became equal to the maternal blood ^{11}C-activity at about 3 hours after dose, i.e., considerably later than was the case for [^{14}C]morphine. No kinetic estimations were made for the ^{11}C-activity curves, since this activity represents the sum of radioactivities of [^{11}C]morphine and metabolites.

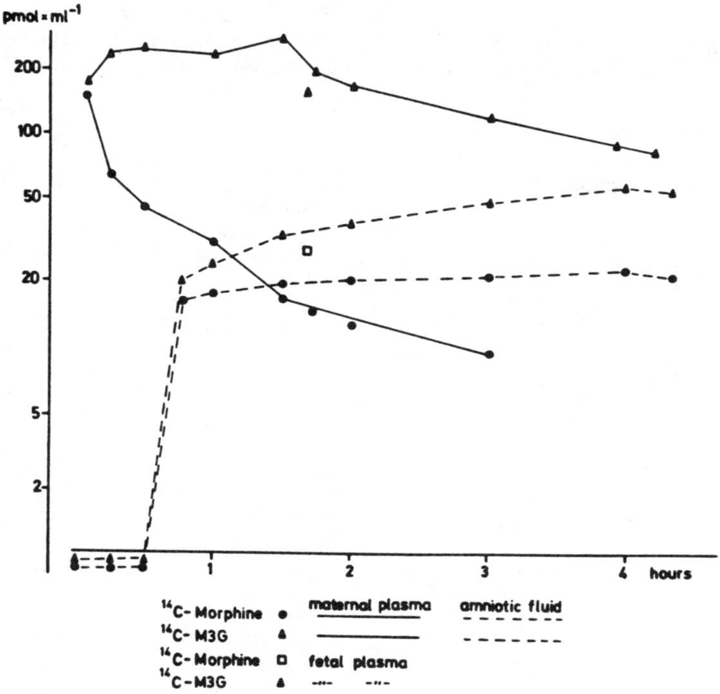

FIGURE 3. [^{14}C]morphine and [^{14}C]morphine-3-glucuronide concentrations in maternal plasma, amniotic fluid, and fetal plasma after administration of [^{14}C]morphine to one monkey.

DISCUSSION

PET has not been used previously for the study of pharmacokinetics in the feto-maternal unit, but it is an accepted technique for studies of brain metabolism and for receptor studies in the brain and heart (Ell and Holman 1982). The advantage of the method for its use during pregnancy is that it is a noninvasive tracer technique, thus avoiding pharmacological effects of administered compounds. The procedure may be repeated within a few hours and performed several times during the pregnancy in the same animal. It is thus suitable for the study of dynamic events during various phases of fetal life.

The use of PET as an in vivo autoradiographic technique gives a unique possibility to study the rapid initial distribution of drugs from mother to fetus.

However, the PET technique has certain shortcomings. The PET image is derived from all molecules labeled with the radionuclide; i.e., both the administered drug and its metabolites. In case the drug is metabolized within 2 hours, blood and urine must be analyzed for the distribution of radioactivity between parent drug and metabolites by chemical analysis, e.g., HPLC. Another approach that facilitates the interpretation of the

PET images is to label the molecule at different sites. The pattern of distribution of the radioactivity when the same individual is investigated with these compounds will give additional information on the metabolism.

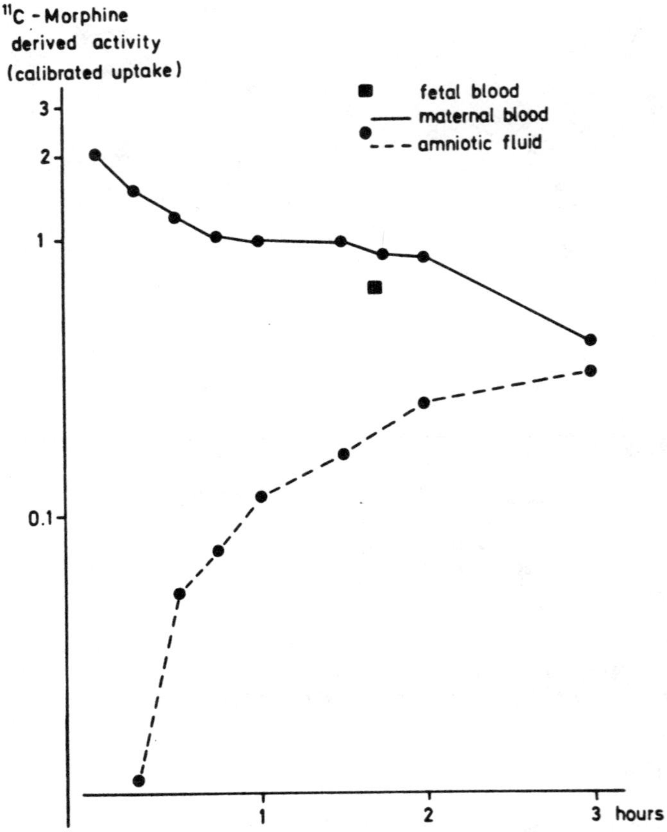

FIGURE 4. [¹¹C]Morphine-derived activity in maternal blood, fetal blood, and amniotic fluid after administration of [¹¹C]morphine to the same monkey as in figure 3.

PET has a fairly low spatial resolution. The distribution of morphine and heroin in the fetal brain is of great interest to study, but we chose to study the liver in our initial experiments. The liver is a homogeneous organ, in which the limited resolution is of less importance than in studies of the central nervous system.

The radioactivity in an organ is composed of two fractions; one is limited to the blood and the other is composed of metabolized and unmetabolized ^{11}C-labeled moieties in the tissues. Corrections for the fraction in the blood pool can be made by a separate determination of the blood volume using ^{11}C-labeled red blood cells or ^{68}Ga-transferrin.

A special difficulty with fetal PET studies is that the fetus might move during the registration even if the mother is immobilized with ketamine. In most cases, however, no difficulties in localizing the fetal liver placenta were experienced.

The short half-life of ^{11}C does not permit observation times exceeding 2 hours. The simultaneous administration of the corresponding unlabeled compound or compounds labeled with long-lived isotopes makes it possible to perform conventional studies with sampling beyond that period. By sampling from the mother and the fetus, the PET image may be correlated to the results from analyses of administered drugs and their metabolites in body fluids. By this combination of techniques, two goals are achieved. First, the initial, rapid phase of transport between different organs of the body is studied by PET. This is not possible by blood sampling alone. Second, results from the analyses of radioactivity and drug concentrations in body fluids may be used in the construction of compartment models. Such models may then be used in future experiments, making invasive sampling techniques necessary only in an initial phase of the study.

The present results indicate that heroin is readily distributed to the fetus in accordance with its high lipophilicity. The transfer rate of morphine was somewhat slower. Our data obtained with ^{14}C-labeled morphine confirm that this drug is transported to the amniotic fluid within 45 minutes. Earlier sampling did not reveal measurable levels of morphine in the fetus. The [^{14}C]M3G/[^{14}C]morphine concentration ratio in maternal blood varied between the monkeys, indicating interindividual variation in the capacity to glucuronidate this drug in the liver (Rane et al. 1984; Säwe et al., in press). This ratio was significantly higher than that in the amniotic fluid at "pseudo-steady-state," which probably reflects the slower passage of the hydrophilic M3G metabolite as compared to the parent drug.

No other method than PET has so far been able to reveal the events within the body without disturbing the integrity of the feto-maternal unit. The ultrasound-guided puncture of the umbilical vein for fetal blood sampling has been without noticeable effect on the animals, but the limiting factor is the volume of blood which can be drawn.

The energy metabolism and the protein synthesis are of great importance for the development of the fetus and, in particular, its central nervous system. Infants of drug-addicted mothers are often small for gestational age. The reasons for this are unknown, but impaired energy utilization and perturbed protein synthesis are possible explanations. Studies of glucose and amino acid transport and metabolism in opiate-treated animals may contribute to the understanding of the causes of this growth retardation.

Another negative effect of drug abuse on the fetus is frequent abstinence symptoms. Our results show that there was a rapid increase in radioactivity in the fetus after intravenous injection of [^{11}C]morphine and [^{11}C]heroin to the mother. The decline of the radioactivity was also rapid, indicating that the fetus may suffer from withdrawal effects. PET has been shown to offer unique possibilities to register such rapid events.

REFERENCES

Bergström, M.; Eriksson, L.; Bohm, C.; Blomqvist, G.; and Litton, J. Correction for scattered radiation in a ring detector positron camera by internal transformation of the projections. J Comput Assist Tomogr 7(1): 42-50, 1983.

Ell, P.J., and Holman, B.L., eds. Computed Emission Tomography Oxford: Oxford University Press, 1982.

Eriksson, L.; Bohm, C.; Kesselberg, M.; Blomqvist, G.; Litton, J.; Widén, L.; Bergström, M.; Ericson, K.; and Greitz, T. A four ring positron camera system for emission tomography in the brain. IEE Trans Nucl Sci 29:539-543, 1982.

Hartvig, P.; Bergström, K.; Lindberg, B.; Lundberg, P.O.; Lundqvist, H.; Långström, B.; Svärd, H.; and Rane, A. Kinetics of ^{11}C-labeled opiates in the brain of rhesus monkeys. J Pharmacol Exp Ther 230:250-255, 1984.

Långström, B.; Antoni, G.; Halldin, C.; Svärd. H.; and Bergson, G. Synthesis of some ^{11}C-labeled alkaloids. Chem Scripta 2:46-48, 1982.

Lindgren, P.G., and Lindberg, B.S. Fetal blood sampling through ultrasound guided puncture of the umbilical vein in rhesus monkeys. J Med Primatol, in press.

Rane, A.; Säwe, J.; Lindberg, B.; Svensson, J.-O.; Garle, M.; Erwald, R.; and Jorulf, H. Morphine glucuronidation in the Rhesus monkeys: A comparative in vivo and in vitro study. J Pharmacol Exp Ther 229:571-576, 1984.

Säwe, J.; Kager, L.; Svensson, J.O. ; and Rane, A. Oral morphine in cancer patients: In vivo kinetics and in vitro hepatic glucuronidation in the individual patients. Br J Clin Pharmacol, in press.

Svensson, J.O.; Rane, A.; Säwe, J.; and Sjöqvist, F. Determination of morphine, morphine-3-glucuronide and (tentatively) morphine-6-glucuronide in plasma and urine using ion-pair high performance liquid chromatography. J Chromatography 230:427-432, 1982.

Wagner, H.; Burns, D.; Dannals, R.; Wong, D.; Långström, B.; Duelfer, T.; Frost, J.; Ravert, H.; Links, J.M.; Rosenblom, S.B.; Lukas, S.; Kramer, A.; and Kuhar, M. Imaging dopamine receptors in the human brain by positron emission tomography. Science 221:1264-1268, 1983.

ACKNOWLEDGMENTS

The study was supported by the Swedish Medical Research Council (14X-04496), The Swedish Cancer Society, and The Expressen Prenatal Research Fund.

AUTHORS

Bo S. Lindberg, M.D., Ph.D.
Department of Obstetrics and Gynecology
University Hospital
751 85 Uppsala, Sweden

Per Hartvig, Pharm.D.
Hospital Pharmacy
University Hospital
751 85 Uppsala, Sweden

Anders Lilja, M.D.
Department of Diagnostic Radiology
University Hospital
751 85 Uppsala, Sweden

Hans Lundqvist, Ph.D.
Department of Physical Biology
Gustaf Werner Institute
University of Uppsala
P.O. 531, 751 21 Uppsala, Sweden

Bengt Långström, Ph.D.
Department of Organic Chemistry
Institute of Chemistry
University of Uppsala
P.O. 531, 751 21 Uppsala, Sweden

Petter Malmborg, M.Sc.
Department of Physical Biology
Gustaf Werner Institute
University of Uppsala
P.O. 531, 751 21 Uppsala, Sweden

Anders Rane, M.D., Ph.D.
Department of Clinical Pharmacology
Huddinge Hospital
Karolinska Institute
141 86 Huddinge, Sweden

Annika Rimland, M.Sc.
Department of Organic Chemistry
Institute of Chemistry
P.O. 531, 751 21 Uppsala, Sweden

Hans Svärd, M.Sc.
Department of Organic Chemistry
P.O. 531, 751 21 Uppsala, Sweden

Placental Transfer of Drugs, Alcohol, and Components of Cigarette Smoke and Their Effects on the Human Fetus

Betty R. Kuhnert and Paul M. Kuhnert

INTRODUCTION

The placenta was once thought to act as a barrier which protected the fetus from the passage of xenobiotic compounds. Now, it is more accurately thought of as a sieve which allows small molecules to pass by diffusion. For example, if the mother smokes, the fetus is exposed to the components of cigarette smoke. Furthermore, if the mother takes drugs, the fetus is exposed to the drugs as well as to any active metabolites. Finally, if the mother drinks alcohol, fetal blood alcohol levels may be similar to those of the mother.

Components of cigarette smoke, alcohol, and other drugs all affect the fetus to varying degrees. These effects can range from subtle neonatal neurobehavioral effects following the use of meperidine during labor to the full teratogenic effects of alcohol known as the fetal alcohol syndrome (FAS). These effects can be short-lived, as in the case of low doses of meperidine given to the mother, or permanent, as in the case of the mental retardation following chronic alcohol use during pregnancy. In some cases, such as exposure to lead or cadmium from cigarette smoke, there may be biological effects, but no obvious clinical effects. In other cases such as alcohol, the lower limits of the teratogenic potential are unknown.

This chapter reviews recent work on the placental transfer of three drugs (meperidine, phencyclidine, and alcohol) and certain components of cigarette smoke (lead, cadmium, and thiocyanate) and examines the effects of these compounds on the fetus.

MEPERIDINE

Meperidine is a synthetic opiate narcotic administered intravenously or intramuscularly for analgesia during labor.

It has been in use since 1939 and today it is the most commonly used obstetrical analgesic (Fishburne 1982). However, despite its widespread use for many years, surprisingly little was known about its pharmacology during the perinatal period.

Some puzzling questions have been raised concerning the use of meperidine during labor. For example, meperidine has been noted to cause respiratory depression in the newborn infant even if given to the mother in low doses (Morrison et al. 1973). Moreover, it has also been shown to cause more neonatal respiratory depression if given to laboring patients 2 to 3 hours prior to delivery rather than 1 hour or less prior to delivery (Guilhem et al. 1953; Shnider and Moya 1964). And, finally, no relationship could be demonstrated between neonatal status and the concentration of meperidine in cord blood (Morrison et al. 1973; Shnider and Moya 1964).

Based on this information, it was hypothesized that the effects of meperidine on neonatal status were due to the formation of a toxic metabolite. Normeperidine was thought to be this active metabolite because animal studies had shown it to be twice as potent as a convulsant and respiratory depressant, but half as potent as meperidine when used as an analgesic (Miller and Anderson 1954). However, the idea of a metabolite reaching the fetus remained a hypothesis because sensitive analytical techniques which could distinguish between meperidine and normeperidine in plasma were not available until the 1970s. Furthermore, it had been reported that neither the pregnant woman nor the neonate could metabolize meperidine to normeperidine (Crawford and Rudofsky 1966).

The mother's ability to demethylate meperidine to normeperidine was recently documented (Kuhnert et al. 1979b). Maternal plasma levels of normeperidine are apparent shortly after injection of the parent drug and levels increase throughout labor. The ratio of normeperidine to meperidine increases steadily with time. Furthermore, normeperidine has been reported in cord blood (Kuhnert et al. 1979a). The levels of normeperidine in cord blood increase with time after injection of the drug in the mother (Kuhnert et al. 1980). With long drug-to-delivery intervals, more normeperidine can be found in cord artery than in cord vein. This reflects uptake of the drug in fetal tissues. Thus, recent studies support the hypothesis of an active meperidine metabolite reaching the fetus. However, the levels of normeperidine following single doses are probably too low to have clinical effects. Moreover, the studies do not explain the increase in neonatal morbidity if delivery occurs 2 to 3 hours after administration of the drug to the mother.

Cord blood levels of drugs at delivery do not necessarily reflect the infant's tissue levels. Since tissue is not available for study from human infants, serial urine collections and calculations of umbilical artery to umbilical vein ratios are used to indirectly estimate tissue equilibrium or body burden of drugs. Using these techniques, it has been shown that maximum uptake of meperidine by fetal tissues occurs 2 to 3 hours after a single intravenous injection of meperidine to the mother (Belfrage et al. 1981; Kuhnert et al. 1979a). Thus, the hypothesis of a toxic metabolite reaching the fetus and causing the neonatal morbidity noted at 2 to 3 hours is not supported. The dose-delivery intervals resulting in maximum uptake of the parent compound, meperidine, correspond with those resulting in maximum neonatal depression.

The use of multiple doses of meperidine over extended time periods during labor may result in concentrations of normeperidine that are high enough to be clinically significant (Kuhnert et al. 1985a; 1985c). In cases of long drug-to-delivery intervals (>4 hours), considerable normeperidine is formed by both mother and fetus (Kuhnert et al. 1985a). Furthermore, following multiple doses, the uptake of meperidine is altered from what occurs following single doses, and the high levels of normeperidine may add to the adverse effects resulting from high levels of the parent compound. Following single doses, maximum tissue uptake of meperidine occurs at 2 to 3 hours following administration of the drug to the mother. After this, there is a diffusion gradient from fetal tissues to fetal blood to maternal blood and the drug is cleared from the fetus. With multiple doses, the diffusion gradient is continuously in the direction of fetal tissue uptake. Thus, continuous uptake of the drug is occurring in fetal tissues for hours after the last dose is given. Therefore, multiple doses of meperidine to the mother over long time periods result in maximum exposure of the fetus to both meperidine and normeperidine (Kuhnert et al. 1985a, 1985c).

There was little doubt that the high levels of meperidine administered to parturients a generation ago could result in neonatal depression (Shnider and Moya 1964). However, obstetricians today use much lower doses and the clinical impression is that there are usually no adverse effects on the neonate. A study designed to test this hypothesis showed that there may be subtle neurobehavioral effects on the fetus due to mean doses as low as 39 ± 19 mg of meperidine to the mother (Kuhnert et al. 1985b). Using the Brazelton Neonatal Behavioral Assessment Scale, it was shown that infants whose mothers received low doses of meperidine performed less well on tests of regulation of state and had more abnormal reflexes than infants of nonmedicated mothers. Furthermore, these effects were related to the drug-to-delivery interval. Performance was less optimal with longer drug to delivery intervals at both 1 and 3 days of life. Since normeperidine levels increase with long drug-to-delivery intervals, and levels of meperidine, but not normeperidine, are very low by 3 days of age, the results of this study again suggest that normeperidine may contribute to the adverse effects following meperidine administration to the mother.

The clinical protocol for the administration of meperidine during labor has changed as more has become known about the pharmacology of the drug in the intrapartum period. It was once suggested that meperidine should be given in 100 to 150 mg doses at hourly intervals up to three doses and then as required (Walker 1973). Today, we know that pharmacologically the best time to be born following intravenous maternal analgesia with meper- idine would be within 1 hour of a single low dose.

PHENCYCLIDINE

Phencyclidine (angel dust) was originally developed as a short acting anesthetic. However, its hallucinogenic effects have limited its legal use to the practice of veterinary medicine. Nevertheless, phencyclidine's sedative and hallucinogenic effects make it a popular drug of abuse among adolescents. These adolescents are often the same ones with unplanned pregnancies.

There has been one isolated report of the possible teratogenic effects of phencyclidine (Golden et al. 1980). However, the use of phencyclidine by pregnant women and possible effects on the fetus have only recently been studied prospectively (Golden et al. 1984). In this study, the frequency of use by pregnant women was estimated to be between 0.8 and 6.4 percent. Most of these women were polydrug users; therefore, the isolated effects of phencyclidine on the fetus are difficult to determine. This study indicated that phencyclidine use during pregnancy was widespread.

Abnormal neonatal neurological and behavioral findings have been associated with maternal phencyclidine exposure (Golden et al. 1985). These findings included poor attention, hypertonic ankle reflex, and depressed neonatal reflexes--grasp and rooting. A second group of abnormal outcomes which were more frequent in study infants, but not statistically different, included miotic pupils, increased brachial reflexes, and decreased joint mobility. The abnormal grasp reflex was predictive of phencyclidine use when stepwise discriminant function analysis was used. Abnormal anatomic findings were not associated with maternal phencyclidine use in this study. These results suggested that phencyclidine exposure to the fetus can result in abnormal neonatal neurologic findings and behavior. Future studies must determine the long-term effects of exposing the fetus to phencyclidine.

The pharmacology of phencyclidine in pregnant women or neonates has not been well studied. Phencyclidine is known to cross the placenta, to be present in neonatal urine and blood, and in breast milk (Strauss et al. 1981; Kaufman et al. 1983a, 1983b). In nonpregnant subjects, phencyclidine is known to be metabolized to two hydroxylated compounds (Lin et al. 1975) and a pentanoic metabolite (Cook et al. 1982). All three metabolites may have pharmacological activity (Domino 1978; Cohen et al. 1982).

The results of analyzing PCP metabolites in spot urine samples collected from asymptomatic pregnant patients suggested that the pentanoic acid metabolite is a major metabolite of PCP in these patients (Kuhnert et al. 1984). This metabolite was present in concentrations many times higher than either the parent compound or the hydroxylated metabolites. However, at delivery the pentanoic acid metabolite did not seem to be the major compound excreted by parturients and this may be due to differences in time since the drug was used. Maternal urine samples were positive for at least 36 hours after delivery and excretion of both drug and metabolites fluctuated.

Phencyclidine and its metabolites have been analyzed in serial samples collected from asymptomatic neonates. The results have shown that excretion of drug and metabolites is erratic and that the samples are positive for at least 36 hours (Kuhnert et al. 1984). Thus, an earlier report that urine is negative after 72 hours in symptomatic infants may have been hampered by insensitive methodology (Strauss et al. 1981). These findings suggest that the drug may have been sequestered in various tissues or body compartments and more detailed pharmacological studies are obviously needed. Furthermore, these results suggest that present methods of screening for phencyclidine use may be inadequate.

ALCOHOL

Historically, alcohol has often been noted to have an adverse effect on offspring. The Bible (Judges 13:7) says: "Behold, thou shalt conceive, and bear a son; and now drink no wine nor strong drink...." In 1973, Jones et al.

recognized a common pattern of malformation in the offspring of alcoholic mothers and called this the fetal alcohol syndrome. Unknown to them, the pattern had already been described in France in 1968 (Lemoine et al.). Since 1973, many more cases of the syndrome have been documented throughout the world (Clarren and Smith 1978; Streissguth et al. 1980).

The principle features of FAS include mental retardation, growth deficiency, and characteristic facial features. These facial features are so characteristic that the mothers can be diagnosed as alcoholics from the children's features alone (Lemoine et al. 1968). These features include small head circumference, low nasal bridge, eyes with prominent epicanthic folds and short palpebral fissures, short nose, indistinct philtrum (groove between nose and mouth), and a thin upper lip. The percentage of infants having the problems associated with the FAS is directly related to the magnitude of maternal ethanol ingestion (Seidenberg and Majewski 1978), and also to the duration of maternal alcoholism (Majewski et al. 1976).

The lower limit of the teratogenic potential of alcohol is unknown. There is now considerable evidence from clinical and experimental studies that prenatal alcohol exposure may adversely affect fetal development; this is true even in the absence of observable physical anomalies and is apparent by behavioral deficits. In addition to lowered IQ, children exhibit various other behavioral problems such as excessive stubbornness, aggression, hyperactivity, and sleep disorders. Furthermore, behavioral anomalies have been reported in neonates of social drinkers (Landesman-Dwyer et al. 1978). In social drinkers who smoked, moderate alcohol intake coupled with moderate smoking use exerted an interactive and deleterious effect upon newborn learning, which was not predictable when the two drugs were taken separately (Martin et al. 1977). Thus, alcohol can be characterized as a potent behavioral teratogen.

There have been relatively few investigations of the disposition of ethanol following maternal administration in humans. Brien et al. (1983) reported that there is a relatively low ethanol concentration in amniotic fluid after maternal administration of ethanol and then a relatively high ethanol concentration in amniotic fluid when ethanol has been virtually eliminated from maternal blood. Hence, the amniotic fluid appears to provide a "chemical cloud" environment such that the fetus remains exposed to ethanol when none is measurable in maternal blood. It is conceivable that, during an episode of binge-type drinking, the fetus could be exposed to a very high ethanol concentration in amniotic fluid for a longer time period than would be predicted by the maternal blood ethanol concentration.

There is no longer any debate that the fetal alcohol syndrome exists (Clarren and Smith 1978). What remains to be answered are such questions as: What is the risk to a woman, given a specific drinking history, of producing a seriously affected offspring? How does intermittent binge drinking as opposed to steady consumption alter the phenotype? How do commonly associated drugs like caffeine, nicotine, and diazepam alter or potentiate the effects of alcohol? What are the mechanisms through which alcohol or its breakdown products produce their effect on the embryo and fetus? And finally, can prenatal diagnostic technics be used to detect this disorder.

SMOKING

Smoking may adversely affect many aspects of human reproduction. For example, it may increase the risk of spontaneous abortion (Himmelberger et al. 1978), retard fetal growth (Meyer et al. 1976), and increase the number of pregnancy complications (Andrews and McGarry 1972). In addition, children of smokers may be physically and intellectually disadvantaged (Goldstein 1971). Precisely why these effects occur is unknown, but many factors are believed to be involved and interrelated. Three such factors may be the increase in the uptake of lead, cadmium, and cyanide which occurs subsequent to exposure to cigarette smoke.

Lead

Each cigarette generates approximately 1 to 2 micrograms of airborne lead when burned (Cogbill and Hobbs 1957). The amount of this lead that reaches the fetus depends on how much the mother smokes. The concentration of lead in fetal blood is directly related to the concentration of lead in maternal blood (Kuhnert et al. 1976). While it is well established that lead is an environmental health hazard to children, its effect on the fetus is not well documented.

The effects of low levels of lead exposure can be seen by looking at the effect of lead on enzymes involved in the pathway of heme synthesis. One of the earliest manifestations of toxicity from low concentration of lead appear to be the inhibition of d-aminolevulinic acid dehydratase (ALAD) which converts d-aminolevulinic acid to porphobilinogen; the other manifestation is ferrochelatase which inserts iron into protoporphyrin IX to form heme. The inhibition of ALAD can be measured directly by enzyme assay (Granick et al. 1973); the inhibition of ferrochelatase can be measured indirectly by increases in erythrocyte protoporphyrin levels (Sassa et al. 1973).

In the fetus there is no relationship between erythrocyte protoporphyrin levels and blood lead at term (Kuhnert et al. 1978). This suggests that there has been no chronic effects of lead in the fetal bone marrow. There is, however, a strong correlation between the erythrocyte lead levels and the activity of ALAD in human fetal erythrocytes (Kuhnert et al. 1977). This suggests that there is a direct acute effect of lead on the enzyme in the peripheral circulation. Enzyme inhibition due to lead averages 11 percent of the enzyme's activity. Infants of smoking mothers were found to have significantly more enzyme inhibition than infants of nonsmoking mothers.

Cadmium

In addition to lead, the average cigarette contains 1 to 2 micrograms of cadmium (Lewis et al. 1972). Heavy smokers may have an intake of 20 micrograms/day or more due to smoking, in addition to intake from dietary sources. In animals, cadmium has been found to cause fetal growth retardation at low concentrations (Webster 1978), and to induce developmental anomalies and fetal death at higher concentrations (Chernoff 1973). In humans, cadmium has been thought to be one of the factors which may contribute to fetal growth retardation (Longo 1980).

Cadmium's adverse biological effects stem from its simularity in molecular structure to the essential element, zinc. Because of this, cadmium can substitute for zinc as a cofactor for several different enzymes, including alcohol dehydrogenase, acid phosphatase, and others. This substitution causes enzyme inhibition. Further biological effects may occur because cadmium in the body is bound to metalothionein, a transport protein which also binds zinc.

The uptake of cadmium by pregnant women who smoke and the disposition of cadmium in the maternal-fetoplacental unit has only recently been described (Kuhnert et al. 1982). A comparison of cadmium levels in maternal blood, fetal blood, and placenta between smokers and nonsmokers showed that the highest concentration of cadmium was found in the placenta of smokers; the least amount was found in the cord blood of infants whose mothers were nonsmokers. The placenta of nonsmokers contained approximately seven times more cadmium than the corresponding cord blood levels; for smokers, this difference was approximately ninefold. Significantly higher cadmium levels were found in maternal blood and placenta of smokers. Cord blood levels were higher, but not significantly, in smokers; the percentage increase in cadmium due to smoking were 16 percent in cord blood, 32 percent in placenta, and 59 percent in maternal blood. It appears from this study and others (Roels et al. 1978; Lauwerys et al. 1978) that the placenta acts as a barrier to the transfer of cadmium to the fetus.

The fact that cadmium does accumulate in the placenta should not be interpreted to mean that exposure to cadmium is not hazardous to the fetus. Accumulation of cadmium in the placenta could alter its function and thus be embryotoxic. It has been shown in animals that the placenta is rapidly damaged after maternal injections of cadmium (Parizek 1965). This leads to embryonic death in utero.

Cyanide

Tobacco smoke also contains cyanide, most of which is rapidly converted to thiocyanate after absorption in the body (Pettigrew and Fell 1972). Although low levels of thiocyanate are normally present in the body from dietary sources, elevations in thiocyanate are believed to be one of the mechanisms of fetal growth retardation related to smoking (Andrews 1973; Pettigrew et al. 1977; Mebert et al. 1979; Pirani 1978). In the body, thiocyanate and cyanide maintain a dynamic equilibrium. In higher doses, thiocyanate and cyanide are definitely toxic. Both can act as hypotensive agents, reduce intracellular oxygen utilization by inhibiting cytochromes, interfere with vitamin B12 metabolism, cause degenerative neurological disease, and alter thyroid function (Andrews 1973; Pettigrew et al. 1977; Mebert et al. 1979; Pirani 1978; Philbrick et al. 1979).

During pregnancy, maternal thiocyanate levels are correlated with the number of cigarettes smoked per day by the mother. Furthermore, maternal and fetal thiocyanate levels are very closely correlated (Pettigrew et al. 1977; Bottoms et al. 1982). Average fetal levels are similar to those in the mother (Bottoms et al. 1982).

Thiocyanate can also be used as an effective biological marker of exposure to smoking (Cohen and Bartsch 1980). This compound is particularly attractive as a marker because of its long half-life (14 days) in the body. Compounds such as carboxyhemoglobin (4 hours) or nicotine (<30 minutes) have much shorter half-lives. One limitation is that the specificity and sensitivity may be inadequate when thiocyanate levels are close to levels due to dietary or other sources. Thiocyanate has recently been used as a biological marker to study the effects of passive smoking on the fetus (Bottoms et al. 1982).

Passive smoking--the exposure of nonsmokers to air contaminated with cigarette smoke--has been suggested as producing some of the same adverse health consequences as active smoking. There are reports of increased frequencies of upper respiratory infection, bronchitis, pneumonia, diminished small airway function, and angina in association with passive smoking in the workplace or in the home (White and Froeb 1980; Tager et al. 1979; Harlap and Davies 1974; Aronow 1978). These findings suggest that passive smoking might also affect the fetus. While there are many studies of active smoking during pregnancy, the effects of passive smoking during pregnancy are not well documented.

Increased fetal thiocyanate has been found in association with passive smoking (Bottoms et al. 1982). This finding suggests that tobacco smoking by other members in the home or workplace of a pregnant woman who does not smoke exposes the fetus to a measurable increase in at least one metabolic byproduct of tobacco smoke, thiocyanate. This is consistent with the possibility that passive smoking might adversely affect the fetus. Unfortunately, there have been no enzymatic or clinical studies to assess possible biological or clinical effects from the relatively small increase in thiocyanate levels associated with passive smoking.

REFERENCES

Andrews J. Thiocyanate and smoking in pregnancy. Br J Obstet Gynaecol 80:810, 1973.

Andrews J., and McGarry, J.M. A community study of smoking in pregnancy. Br J Obstet Gynaecol 79:1057, 1972.

Aronow, W.S. Effect of passive smoking on angina pectoris. N Engl J Med 299:21, 1978.

Belfrage, P.; Boreus, L.O.; Hartvig, P.; Irestedt, L.; and Raabe, N. Neonatal depression after obstetrical analgesia with pethidine. The role of the injection-delivery time interval and of the plasma concentrations of pethidine and norpethidine. Acta Obstet Gynecol Scand 60:43, 1981.

Bottoms, S.F.; Kuhnert, B.R.; Kuhnert, P.M.; and Reese, A.L.P. Maternal passive smoking and fetal serum thiocyanate levels. Am J Obstet Gynecol 144:787, 1982.

Brien, J.F.; Loomis, C.W.; Tranmer, J.; and McGrath, M. Disposition of ethanol in human maternal venous blood and amniotic fluid. Am J Obstet Gynecol 146:181, 1983.

Chernoff, N. Teratogenic effects of cadmium in rats. Teratology 8:29, 1973.

Clarren, S.K., and Smith, D.W. The fetal alcohol syndrome. N Engl J Med 298:1063, 1978.

Cogbill, E.C., and Hobbs, M.E. Transfer of metallic constituents of cigarettes to the main-stream smoke. Tobacco 144(19):24, 1957.

Cohen, J.D., and Bartsch, G.E. A comparison between carboxyhemoglobin and serum thiocyanate determinations as indicators of cigarette smoking. Am J Public Health 70:284, 1980.

Cohen, L.S.; Gosenfeld, L.; Wilkins, J.; Krammerer, R.C.; and Tachiki, K. Demonstration of an amino acid metabolite of phencyclidine. N Engl J Med 306:1472, 1982.

Cook, C.E.; Brine, D.R.; Jeffcoat, A.R.; Hill, J.M.; Wall, M.E.; Perez-Reyes, M.; and DiGuiseppi, S.R. Phencyclidine disposition after intravenous and oral doses. Clin Pharmacol Ther 31:625, 1982.

Crawford, J.S., and Rudofsky, S. Some alterations in the pattern of drug metabolism associated with pregnancy, oral contraception, and the newlyborn. Br J Anaesthesiol 38:446, 1966.

Dominio, E.F. Neurobioilogy of phencyclidine: An update. In: Petersen, R.C., and Stillman, R.C., eds. Phencyclidine Abuse: An Appraisal. National Institute on Drug Abuse Research Monograph 21. DHEW Pub No. (ADM) 78-728. Washington, D.C.: Supt. of Docs., U.S. Govt. Print. Off., 1978. pp. 18-43.

Fishburne, J.I. Systemic analgesia during labor. Clinics in Perinatol 9(10):29, 1982.

Golden, N.L.; Sokol, R.J.; and Rubin, I.L. Angel dust: Possible effects on the fetus. Pediatrics 65(1):18, 1980.

Golden, N.L.; Kuhnert, B.R.; Sokol, R.J.; Martier, S. and Bagby, B.S. Phencyclidine use during pregnancy. Am J Obstet Gynecol 148(3):254, 1984.

Golden, N.L.; Kuhnert, B.R.; Sokol, R.J.; Martier, S.; and Williams, T. neonatal manifestations of maternal phencyclidine exposure. Submitted to Am J Obstet Gynecol, 1985.

Goldstein, H. Factors influencing the height of seven year old children: Results from the national child development study. Hum Biol 43:92, 1971.

Granick, J.L.; Sassa, S.; Granick, S.; Levere, R.D.; and Kappas, A. Studies in lead poisoning. II: Correlation between ratio of activated to inactivated delta aminolevulinic acid dehydratase of whole blood and the blood lead level. Biochem Med 8:149, 1973.

Guilhem, P.; Pentonnier, A.; Baux, R.; Bourbon, P.; and Bennet, P. Les effects sur le nouveau-né de la péthidine. Gynecol Obstet 52(2):196, 1953.

Harlap, S., and Davies, A.M. Infant admissions to hospital and maternal smoking. Lancet 1:529, 1974.

Himmelberger, D.V.; Brown, B.W., Jr.; and Cohen, E.N. Cigarette smoking during pregnancy and the occurrence of spontaneous abortion and congenital abnormality. Am J Epidemiol 108:470, 1978.

Jones, K.L.; Smith, D.W.; Ulleland, C.N.; and Streissguth, A.P. Pattern of malformation in offspring of chronic alcoholic mothers. Lancet 1:1267, 1973.

Kaufman, K.R.; Petrucha, R.A.; Pitts, F.N.; and Weekes, J.D. PCP in amniotic fluid and breast milk: case report. J Clin Psychol 44(7):269, 1983a.

Kaufman, K.R.; Petruchua, R.A.; Pitts, F.N.; and Kaufman, E.R. Phencyclidine in umbilical cord blood: Preliminary data. Am J Psychol 140(4):450, 1983b.

Kuhnert, B.R.; Kuhnert, P.M.; Tu, A.S.L.; Lin, D.C.K.; and Foltz, R.L. Meperidine and normeperidine levels following meperidine administration during labor. I. Mother. Am J Obstet Gynecol 133(8):904, 1979a.

Kuhnert, B.R.; Kuhnert, P.M.; Tu, A.S.L.; and Lin, D.C.K. Meperidine and normeperidine levels following meperidine administration during labor. II. Fetus and neonate. Am J Obstet Gynecol 133(8):909, 1979b.

Kuhnert, B.R.; Kuhnert, P.M.; and Knapp, D.R. Relationship between cord vein normeperidine and time. Am J Obstet Gynecol, Letter to the Editor 137:4, 1980.

Kuhnert, B.R.; Golden, N.L.; Syracuse, C.D.; Bagby, B.S.; and Kuhnert, P.M. Phencyclidine disposition in mother and neonate. Res Comm Sub Abuse 5(3):187, 1984.

Kuhnert, B.R.; Kuhnert, P.M.; Philipson, E.H.; and Syracuse, C.D. Disposition of meperidine and normeperidine following multiple doses during labor. II. Fetus and neonate. Am J Obstet Gynecol 151:410, 1985a.

Kuhnert, B.R.; Linn, P.L.; Kennard, M.J.; and Kuhnert, P.M. Effects of low doses of meperidine on neonatal behavior. Anesth Anal 64:335, 1985b.

Kuhnert, B.R.; Philipson, E.H. Kuhnert, P.M.; and Syracuse, C.D. Disposition of meperidine and normeperidine following multiple doses during labor. I. Mother. Am J Obstet Gynecol 151:406, 1985c.

Kuhnert, P.M.; Kuhnert, B.R.; and Erhard, P. Effect of lead on delta-aminolevulinic acid dehydratase activity in maternal and fetal erythrocytes. In: Hemphill, D.D. ed. Trace Substances in Environmental Health-X. A Symposium. Columbia: University of Missouri, 1976. pp. 373-381.

Kuhnert, P.M.; Erhard, P.; and Kuhnert, B.R. Lead and aminolevulinic acid dehydratase in RBC's of urban mothers and fetuses. Environ Res 14:73-80, 1977.

Kuhnert, P.M.; Erhard, P.; and Kuhnert, B.R. Lead, protoporphyrin, and d-alad levels in human fetal erythrocytes. In: Kirchgessner, M., ed. Trace Element Metabolism in Man and Animals - III, 1978. pp. 593-596.

Kuhnert, P.M.; Kuhnert, B.R.; Erhard, P; and Bottoms, S.F. Cadmium levels in maternal blood, fetal cord blood, and placental tissues of pregnant women who smoke. Am J Obstet Gynecol 142(8): 1021, 1982.

Landesman-Dwyer, S.; Keller, S.L.; and Streissguth, A.P. Naturalistic observations of newborns: Effects of maternal alcohol intake. Alcoholism: Clin and Exper Res 2(2):171, 1978.

Lauwerys, R.; Buchet, J.P.; Roels, H.; and Hubermont, G. Placental transfer of lead, mercury, cadmium, and carbon monoxide in women. I. Comparison of the frequency distributions of the biological indices in maternal and umbilical cord blood. Environ Res 15:278, 1978.

Lemoine, P.; Harousseau, H.; Borteyru, J.P.; and Menuet, J. Les enfants de parents alcoliques: Anomalies observees. Ouest Med 25:476, 1968.

Lewis, G.P.; Jusko, W.J.; and Coughlin, L.L. Cadmium accumulation in man: Influence of smoking, occupation, alcoholic habit and disease. J Chronic Dis 25(12):717, 1972.

Lin, D.C.K.; Fentiman, A.F.; Foltz, R.L.; Forney, R.D.; and Sunshine, I. Quantification of phencyclidine in body fluids by gas chromatography chemical ionization mass spectrometry and identification of two metabolites. Biomed Mass Spectrom 2:206, 1975.

Longo, L.D. Environmental pollution and pregnancy: Risks and uncertainties for the fetus and infant. Am J Obstet Gynecol 137:162, 1980.

Majewski, F.; Bierich, J.R.; Loser, H.; Michaelis, R.; Lieber, B.; and Bettecken, F. On the diagnosis and pathogenesis of alcohol embryopathy (Report on 68 patients). Muench Med Wochenschr 118:1635, 1976.

Martin, J.; Martin, D.C.; and Lund, C.A. Maternal alcohol ingestion and cigarette smoking and their effects on newborn conditioning. Alcoholism: Clin and Exper Res 1(3):243, 1977.

Mebert, A.; Sande, H.; Foss, O.P.; and Stenwig, J.T. Smoking during pregnancy - Effects on the fetus and on thiocyanate levels in mother and baby. Acta Paediatr Scand 68:547, 1979.

Meyer, M.G.; Jonas, B.S.; and Tonascia, J.A. Perinatal events associated with maternal smoking during pregnancy. Am J Epidemiol 103:464, 1976.

Miller, J.W., and Anderson H.H. The effect of N-demethylation on certain pharmacologic actions of morphine, codeine, and meperidine in the mouse. J Pharmacol Exp Ther 112:191, 1954.

Morrison, J.C.; Wiser, W.L.; Rosser, S.I.; Gayden, J.D.; Bucovaz, E.T.; Whybrew, W.D.; and Fish, S.A. Metabolites of meperidine related to fetal depression. Am J Obstet Gynecol 115(8):1132, 1973.

Parizek, J. The peculiar toxicity of cadmium during pregnancy. An experimental "toxemia of pregnancy" induced by cadmium salts. J Reprod Fertil 9:111, 1965

Pettigrew, A.R., and Fell, G.S. Simplified colorimetric determination of thiocyanate in biological fluids, and its application to investigation of the toxic amblyopias. Clin Chem 18:996, 1972.

Pettigrew, A.T.; Logan, R.W.; and Willocks, J. Smoking in pregnancy--Effects on birthweight and on cyanide and thiocyanate levels in mother and baby. Br J Obstet Gynaecol 84:31, 1977.

Philbrick, O.G.; Hopkins, J.B.; Hill, O.C.; Alexander, J.C.; and Thomson, R.G. Effects of prolonged cyanide and thiocyanate feeding in rats. J Toxicol Environ Health 5:579, 1979.

Pirani, B.B.K. Smoking during pregnancy. Obstet Gynecol Surv 33:1, 1978.

Roels, H.; Hubermont, G.; Buchet, J.P.; and Lauwerys, R. Placental transfer of lead, mercury, cadmium, and carbon monoxide in women. III. Factors influencing the accumulation of heavy metals in the placenta and the relationship between metal concentration in the placenta and in maternal and cord blood. Environ Res 16:236, 1978.

Sassa, S.; Granick, J.L.; Granick, S.; Kappas, A.; and Levere, R.D. Studies in lead poisoning. I.: Microanalysis of erythrocyte protoporphyrin levels by spectrofluorometry in detection of chronic lead intoxication in the subclinical range. Biochem Med 8:135, 1973.

Seidenberg, J., and Majewski, F. Frequency of alcohol embryopathy in the different phases of maternal alcoholism. Suchtgefahren 24:63–75, 1978.

Shnider, S.M., and Moya, F. Effects of meperidine on the newborn infant. Am J Obstet Gynecol 89(8):1009, 1964.

Strauss, A.A.; Modanlow, H.D.; and Bosu, S.K. Neonatal manifestations of maternal phencyclidine (PCP) abuse. Pediatrics 68(4):550, 1981.

Streissguth, A.P.; Landesman-Dwyer, S.; Martin, J.C.; and Smith, D.W. teratogenic effects of alcohol in humans and laboratory animals. Science 209:353, 1980.

Tager, I.B.; Weiss, S.T.; Rosner, B.; and Speizer, F.D. Effect of parental cigarette smoking on the pulmonary function of children. Am J Epidemiol 110:15, 1979.

Walker, P.A. Drugs used in labour: An obstetrician's view. Br J Anaesth 45:787, 1973.

Webster, W.S. Cadmium-induced fetal growth retardation in the mouse. Arch Environ Health 33:36, 1978.

White, J.R., and Froeb, H. F. Small airway dysfunction in nonsmokers chronically exposed to tobacco smoke. N Engl J Med 302:720, 1980.

ACKNOWLEDGMENTS

Supported in part by National Institutes of Health, United States Public Health Service grants 5M01-RR00210, N01-RR-8-2112, R01-HD-13359, and R01-DAU-2903.

AUTHORS

Betty R. Kuhnert, Ph.D.
Paul M. Kuhnert, Ph.D.
Perinatal Clinical Research Center
Cleveland Metropolitan General Hospital
Case Western Reserve University
3395 Scranton Road
Cleveland, Ohio 44109

Appendix
Maternal-Fetal Transfer of Abused Substances: Pharmacokinetic and Pharmacodynamic Data

Charles C. Lee and C. Nora Chiang

The objective of this appendix is to present pharmacokinetic and pharmacodynamic data in a format that allows the investigators to readily review research findings regarding pre- and post-natal effects due to maternal exposure to substances of abuse. It is intended to be a comprehensive collection of clinical reports from human studies and laboratory findings in animals as well as perfused placenta preparations. Information on the experimental method, dosage to the mother, route of drug administration, gestational age, and the duration of maternal/fetal exposure is also presented. The abused substances compiled in this appendix include: amphetamines, cannabinoids/delta-9-tetrahydrocannabinol (THC)/cannabis, cocaine, lysergic acid diethylamide (LSD), meperidine, methadone/acetylmethadol, morphine/heroin, nicotine/tobacco, and phencyclidine (PCP).

The pharmacokinetic data in this appendix, where available in the mother and fetus, include half-life ($t_{1/2}$), clearance (Cl), and time to peak concentration (t_{max}). In most cases, the maternal to fetal concentration ratio of drug in the tissue or biological fluid is reported because serial blood sampling required for pharmacokinetic study is not feasible in small animals. Since drug secretion in human breast milk is a critical concern for breast-feeding mothers, information on this subject is also documented for its important clinical implications.

The pharmacodynamic data encompass the broadly defined teratological effects. Traditionally, the term teratology refers to the study of congenital malformations produced by exogenous agents during gestation. In recent years, teratologists have extended their observations beyond morphological changes and have focused on functional disorders for drug-induced biochemical and behavioral anomalies detected at birth or later. Teratological effects for a specific abused substance are documented and compared between animal species.

In the past decade, several tables of pharmacodynamic data for various drug substances have been published. In 1976, Coyle et al. published a review on behavioral teratogenesis in which they summarized prenatal drug effects on behavior as a function of developmental stage. Of the drugs examined, only THC and amphetamine belong to traditionally defined substances of abuse. In 1977, Joneja presented a thorough study on the teratologic effects of THC, given orally as single and multiple doses during gestation, on the fetuses of golden syrian hamsters. Extensive observations were made on day 15 after drug administration, among which were percent resorption or death, number of retarded fetus and external/skeletal abnormalities. No kinetic data were presented. In 1980, Slone et al. tabulated in a symposium proceedings some embryonically toxic drugs and chemicals of potential risk to the human fetus and newborn, recording the number of cases studied and the elicited teratologic effects. In the same year, Abel compiled two tables documenting prenatal effects of cannabis extract and THC. These tables include information about dosage, route of administration, duration of drug exposure during gestation, and teratological effects. Again, no kinetic data were included in the compilation. Until very recently, only data on the effects of pregnancy on drug pharmacokinetics were compiled. Information on the fetal cord to maternal plasma ratio of drug concentrations and drug excretion in human breast milk were compiled as two tables by Parker (1984) for some 60 drugs, most of which were not substances of abuse. Since Parker's review focused on kinetic information, those dynamic effects incurred as a result of placental drug transfer were not documented. An overview of this research area indicates that very little integrated kinetic/dynamic information has been documented. Thus, this compilation is intended to integrate pharmacokinetic and pharmacodynamic data relevant to maternal-fetal transfer of abused substances. It is hoped that this information will add to our understanding and appreciation of this critical subject matter.

Several considerations were given in compiling the following list: (1) Only values obtained from original papers, dating from 1974, and with data or experimental methods which we could evaluate are included. Two review articles for LSD are included because extensive research was performed before that year. (2) The drug must be historically or currently abused to a significant extent. Alcohol and benzodiazepines are not included in this review since there exists such extensive literature on these subjects that separate reviews would be required. (3) Information on dosage, route of administration, and gestational age was lacking in some case studies, particularly when human abusers were involved. However, we feel that kinetic and dynamic effects elicited in pregnant women are sufficiently important to warrant documentation of such effects even without accurate recording of drug dosage regimen. (4) Some duplicate studies using the same animal model and drug are included for the purpose of contrasting the inter-laboratory variation of kinetic/dynamic effects. Apparent deviations in dosage, route of administration, gestational age, and duration of exposure are indicated. (5) The references are keyed to individual authors so that readers can readily locate the reference actually used.

It would obviously be most useful if there were a consensus about the correct value for a given pharmacokinetic parameter or pharmacodynamic measurement in a given species. In this compilation, a single value from the literature or a range of values was selected for each parameter/measurement. In some cases, we have summarized and interpreted the data from the literature to determine the values reported in this table.

We hope that this compilation will serve as a comprehensive reference to those research scientists faced with selection of animal models for drug abuse research in pregnancy. For the general public concerned with the clinical consequences of maternal-fetal transfer of abused substances, this compilation may be appreciated as a warning, particularly for potential drug abusers.

Model/ Preparation	Dose/Route/Time of Exposure	Kinetic/Dynamic Effects	Reference
Drug Category: AMPHETAMINE/METHAMPHETAMINE			
Human	237 out of 42,101 pregnancies used d-amphetamine for control of wt gain during pregnancy	4% reduction in birth wt when drug was taken after 28 wk of gestation; no effects on birth lengths, head circumferences, and perinatal mortality rates	Naeye 1983
Human	amphetamine-addicted women; gr 1: discontinued during first trimester; gr 2: throughout pregnancy	rate of preterm delivery and perinatal motality increased for gr 2	Eriksson et al. 1981
Human	amphetamine-addicted women; gr 1: discontinued during first trimester; gr 2: throughout pregnancy; gr 3: throughout pregnancy & children in foster home	temporary drowsiness in the infants during the first month after birth, normal somatic and psychomotor development at the age of 12 months; symptoms indicating emotional disturbance were common in gr 2	Billing et al. 1980
Human	amphetamines or other anorectic drugs for wt control during pregnancy	no effect on severe congenital anomaly (SCA) rate for live-born children at 5, an excess of oral clefts in the offspring of mother who took amphetamine during early pregnancy	Milkovich & van den Berg 1977

Rat	0, 3 mg/kg/d, bid, d-amphetamine, SC, d 7 thru 20 of gestation	either-way avoidance learning in the offspring was affected; pre- and post-natal amphetamine effects on avoidance behavior dependent on nature of the response and genetic lines	Satinder & Sterling 1983
Rat	0, 0.5 mg/kg/d, dl-amphetamines, SC, during pregnancy	significant decrease in brain alpha but not beta adrenergic receptor binding without apparent changes in receptor affinity in the adult offspring	Ramirez et al. 1983
Rat	0, 2 mg/kg/d, d-amphetamine, SC, d 7 of gestation till birth	offspring showed marked alterations in brain neurotransmitter metabolism, enhanced locomotor activity until 21 days of age	Bigl et al. 1982
Rat	0, 0.5, 1, 2 mg/kg/d, d-amphetamine, SC, d 12 to 15 of gestation	no detectable maternal or fetal toxicity; significant deficit in Y-maze performance, & increased locomotor responsiveness to postnatal challenge of amphetamine in the juvenile offspring	Adams et al. 1982
Rat	0, 2, 5 mg/kg/d, d-amphetamine mixed with drinking water, 30 d prior to mating till parturition	delayed eye & vagina openings, slower in behavioral tests of righting reflexes before 6 days of age and of bridgecrossing at 14 days of age; no differences in open-field activity	Monder 1981
Rat	0, 5 mg/kg/d, methamphetamine; 3 mg/kg/d nicotine; bid, SC, throughout pregnancy & nursing	increased locomotor activity in offspring of methamphetamine-treated group when monitored one night/month from 3-39 months of age	Martin & Martin 1981

Model/ Preparation	Dose/Route/Time of Exposure	Kinetic/Dynamic Effects	Reference
Rat	0, 0.5 mg/kg/d, dl-amphetamine, SC, throughout pregnancy	sexual behavior responses to ovarian steroids were affected for female offspring; no differences in hypothalamic monoamine content, sex cycle duration, and ovulatory phenomena	Ramirez et al. 1979
Rat	0, 5 mg/kg/d, methamphetamine; 3 mg/kg/d, nicotine; SC, or no injection, throughout pregnancy & nursing	increased susceptibility to disease, or possible greater susceptibility to tumor formation and growth retardation for much of the lifespan of offspring of methamphetamine group	Martin et al. 1979
Rat	1.25 mg/kg/d, N-2-cyanoethylamphetamine, PO, d 5 to 21 of pregnancy	increased total lipid content in fetal heart but no differences in lipids in placenta and fetal liver	Kulay et al. 1978
Rat	0, 0.5 mg/kg/d, dl-amphetamine, SC, throughout pregnancy	no modifications of brain endogeneous content of dopamine and noradrenaline but modifications of catecholamine metabolism	Nasello & Ramirez 1978a
Rat	0, 0.5 mg/kg/d, dl-amphetamine, SC, throughout pregnancy	higher motor activity in the open-field test in adults, more errors observed in the Lashley III maze in the first 4 days of age	Nasello & Ramirez 1978b

Rat	0, 5 mg/kg/d, methamphetamine; 3 mg/kg/d nicotine; SC, or no injection, throughout pregnancy & nursing	offspring of methamphetamine gr were significantly underweight, exhibited developmental delay, greater activity for 8 of the first 12 monthly assessments begun at 90 days of age	Martin et al. 1976
Rat	1 or 3 mg/kg, d-amphetamine, bid, SC, from d 5 of gestation till term	no obvious teratogenic effects but a significant and dose-related increase in pup mortality; surviving offspring of 3 mg/kg gr showed increased motor activity and decreased brain biogenic amine levels	Hitzemann et al. 1976
Rat	0, 5, or 10 mg/kg/d d-amphetamine, SC, during d 5-9 (early) or 12-16 (late) of gestation	no differences among offspring in mild expression of emotionality; increased incidences of severe emotional responses (wild running and convulsion) in placebo-early group	Seliger 1975
Rat	0, 1, 3, 5 mg/kg, bid, methamphetamine, throughout gestation	earlier delivery, decreased wt gain over gestation, litter size decreased as a function of dose, eye opening delayed, no gross anomalities, more conditioned avoidance responses for 5 mg/kg group	Martin 1975
Rat	0, 0.5 mg/kg/d, dl-amphetamine, SC, throughout pregnancy	no differences in the age of eyes or vaginal aperture, or in the rate of growth; better acquisition & retention of conditioned avoidance response at the age of 90 days, and lower hippocampal seizure threshold	Nasello et al. 1974

Model/ Preparation	Dose/Route/Time of Exposure	Kinetic/Dynamic Effects	Reference
Mouse	5 mg/kg, ^{3}H-d-amphetamine, IP, on d 16 of gestation	T_{max}=1 hr in placenta & fetal tissues, T_{max}=15 min in matured tissues, conc in fetal tissues lower than maternal tissues	Shah and Yates 1978
Mouse	0, 5 mg/kg/d d-amphetamine, IP, during the last 6-7 d of pregnancy	slightly reduced body wht at birth, altered conc of brain catecholamines during development and increased activity after they had matured	Middaugh et al. 1974
Drug Category: CANNABINOIDS/DELTA-9-TETRAHYDROCANNABINOL(THC)/CANNABIS			
Human	daily smoking of marijuana in third trimester of pregnancy	THC in maternal blood was 2.5-6 times greater than in cord blood; maternal level of metabolite was 4-7 times higher than cord level	Blackard & Tennes 1984
Human	use of marijuana during pregnancy	more meconium staining and longer duration of labor	Greenland et al. 1982
Human	nursing mothers smoking marijuana	THC conc in milk was higher than that in maternal plasma; THC was absorbed by the baby from the milk	Perez-Reyes 1982
Human	use of marijuana during pregnancy	nervous system abnormalities in infants; visual responses were affected in a dose-related manner	Fried 1980

Monkey	2.4 mg/kg/d, PO, throughout pregnancy & lactation	infants showed an alteration in visual attention	Golub et al. 1982
Monkey	2.4 mg/kg/d, IV, during gestation and nursing period	drug-exposed mother-infant pairs were similar to nontreated controls; adequate maternal care was demonstrated by all mothers	Golub et al. 1981
Sheep	0.5 mg/kg, pulmonary infusion 131-140 d of gestation	decreased cardiac output, increased blood pressure, and increased uterine blood flow in mothers; decreased fetal blood pressure, increased umbilical blood flow in fetus; both mother and fetus developed acidosis and hypoxemia	Cotterill et al. 1984
Dog	0.5 mg/kg, IV, 58-63 d of gestation	THC level in maternal brain was 3 times higher than that in fetal brain; major area of THC distribution remained the same	Martin et al. 1977
Rabbit	15, 30, 60 mg/kg/d, SC, 7-19 d of gestation	reduction in maternal food consumption and wt gain, embryotoxicity and embryocidal effects	Sofia et al. 1979
Rabbit/ Rat	0.5-5 mg/kg PO as THC, 5-50 mg/kg PO as crude extract, 6-18 d of gestation	no evidence of teratogenic activity; fetal and pup survival was reduced only at high dose (50 mg/kg of crude marijuana extract)	Wright et al. 1976
Hamster	125-500 mg/kg single dose, 25-100 mg/kg multiple dose, 7-12 d of gestation	higher frequency of fetal mortality and growth retardation, no clearcut teratogenic response	Joneja 1977

Model/ Preparation	Dose/Route/Time of Exposure	Kinetic/Dynamic Effects	Reference
Rat	5-50 mg/kg/d, PO, from pregnancy to d 5 of gestation, then either 50 or 150 mg/kg/d till 21 d of gestation	dose-related decrease in pregnancies carried to term, decrease in wt gain during pregnancy, decrease in birth wt	Abel 1984
Rat	20-200 mg/kg marijuana extract intubation throughout gestation	reduced food-water consumption, reduced maternal wt gain, decreased pup wt at birth, increased mortality	Abel et al. 1981
Rat	4.2 mg/kg/d, IP, 2-6 d of gestation	pups having lower body wt, higher emotionality, poor learning capacity	Kawash et al. 1980
Rat	1-10 mg/kg, PO, during gestation & lactation	small doses THC suppressed luteinizing hormone, larger doses elevated follicle-stimulating hormone and estrogens	Rosencrantz & Esber 1980
Rat	10-150 mg/kg/d marijuana extract intubation 1-21 d of gestation	impaired rotarod performance but did not affect inclined plane, spontaneous alteration, learning/memory, or open-field performance	Abel 1979
Rat	3.3 mg/d, inhalation 1-19 d of gestation	smaller infants at birth, delayed physiological development and less active than the control group	Fried & Charlebois 1979

Rat	1.25 or 4.0 mg/kg, IV, during nursing period	THC inhibited suckling-induced prolactin release in the postpartum rat	Bromley et al. 1978
Rat	2 mg/kg/d, PO, throughout pregnancy	no teratogenicity, but had passive avoidance response	Vardaris 1976
Rat	25, 50, 100 mg/kg/d, SC, 6-15 d of gestation	maternal wt gain depressed, fetal wt decreased significantly at dose greater than 50 mg/kg; some abnormalities	Banerjie et al. 1975
Rat/ Mouse	rat: 12.5-50 mg/kg, PO mouse: 150-600 mg/kg, PO 6-15 d of gestation	no severe sign of intoxication in both rats and mice; increased litter resorption & fetal mortality	Fleischman et al. 1980
Mouse	50 mg THC, single oral dose on 18th d of gestation	maternal exposure altered endocrine function and conc of brain biogenic amines in the male offspring	Dalterio et al. 1984a
Mouse	50 mg/kg, single oral dose on the day of delivery	maternal exposure altered male reproductive function and brain biogenic amines in male and female offspring	Dalterio et al. 1984b
Mouse	20 mg/kg, PO, 3 times/wk 3 wk after weaning & prior to parturition	decreased nest-building behavior, litter size, and sexual behavior	Frischknecht et al. 1982
Mouse	50 mg/kg/d, PO, THC, 12th d of gestation for 4 days	maternal exposure resulted in increase of body wt, ano-genital distance, and testosterone conc in male and female fetuses	Dalterio & Bartke 1981
Mouse	50 mg/kg/d, PO for 7 days from 20th d of gestation	reduced postnatal viability, impaired male reproductive behavior at maturity and decreased seminal vesicle wt	Hatoum et al. 1981

Model/ Preparation	Dose/Route/Time of Exposure	Kinetic/Dynamic Effects	Reference
Mouse	50 mg/kg/d, PO, 1 d prior to parturition and 6 d postpartum	reduced testes wt and elevated plasma level of luteinizing hormone	Dalterio 1980
Mouse	5 mg/kg, PO, during lactation	decrease of pup body wt, some effects on tail length, projection of ears, & eyes opening	Frischknecht et al. 1980
Mouse	0-25 mg/kg/d intubation short term: 8 d long term: 70 d	short term: delayed entry into proestrus, depressed serum progesterone during luteal phase, inhibited female receptivity to males long term: term pregnancies were reduced, no significant effects on length of estrous cycles or mating	Kostellow et al. 1980
Mouse	25 mg/kg/d, SC, from 13th d of pregnancy to term	THC suppressed mammary gland lipoprotein lipase activity and depressed mammary gland growth and development	Raine et al. 1978
Mouse	3-400 mg/kg, single dose, IV, SC, & intragastric	fetal growth retardation, increased external abnormalities, skeletal abnormalities	Joneja 1976
Mouse	50-300 mg/kg, IP, 8-16 d of gestation	in utero death, reduction of body size, offspring with cleft palate	Mantilla-Plata, & Harbison 1976

Mouse	5-150 mg/kg, PO, 6-15 d of gestation	no effects on maternal wt gain, prenatal mortality, fetal wt, and frequency of gross external, internal, & skeletal abnormalities	Fleischman et al. 1975
Drug Category: COCAINE			
Rat/Mouse	50, 60, 75 mg/kg, IP, 8-12 d of gestation	rat: reduction in maternal and fetal wt, increased resorption frequency mouse: decreased fetal wt with no increase in malformations	Fantel & Macphail 1982
Mouse	75-175 mg/kg, SC, 7-12 d of gestation	eye and skeletal defects, teratogenic and ontogenic	Mahalik et al. 1980
Mouse	10 mg/kg ^{3}H-cocaine IP, 15-17 d of gestation	Significant levels of cocaine in placenta and the fetus	Shah et al. 1980
Human Placenta	280-560 umole, cocaine incubate with placenta villi for 10-15 min	decreased acetylcholine release rate by 33-50%	Sastry et al. 1977
Drug Category: LYSERGIC ACID DIETHYLAMIDE (LSD)			
Human	parents used LSD before and during pregnancy	an infant with a unilateral anophthalmia and normal chromosome	Margolis & Martin 1980
Human	maternal LSD use during the first trimester	a premature baby with severe ocular malformations	Chan et al. 1978
Human	Maternal LSD use before & during pregnancy	baby with multiple systemic and ocular malformations	Apple and Bennett 1974

Model/ Preparation	Dose/Route/Time of Exposure	Kinetic/Dynamic Effects	Reference
Human	psychotherapeutic management before pregnancy	no cytogenetic abnormality for mothers and infants	Fernandez et al. 1974
Human	5 psychiatric patients treated with LSD during pregnancy	no abnormal births in 7 pregnancies	Robinson et al. 1974
Human	140 women used LSD before & during pregnancy (polydrug users)	out of 148 pregnancies, 83 live newborns and 8 with major defects, 53 therapeutic abortions, 12 spontaneous abortions	Jacobson & Berlin 1972
Human/ Animals	a review article	five out of 161 children with limb defects but no strong evidence of chromosome breakage and teratogenicity in animals or man	Long 1972
Human/ Animals	a review article	no evidence that pure LSD is teratogenic in humans; some indication of an increased risk of spontaneous abortion in humans; teratogenic effects reported but not confirmed in hamsters and rats, suggested for lower primates and confirmed in mice.	Dishotsky et al. 1971
Rabbit	0, 50 ug/kg, IV, single dose, at 21-25 d of gestation	induced a disaggregation of polysomes in fetal kidney, liver, and brain; pretreatment with haloperidol and pizotyline effectively inhibited the disaggregation	Heikkila et al. 1979

483-942 O - 85 - 5 : QL 3

Rat	^{3}H-LSD, 24 uCi/kg, IV, 18 d of gestation	significant fraction of the dose appeared in the fetus	Back & Singh 1977
Mouse	5 ug/kg, IP, on post-conception d 12 or 18	variable changes in the wt of some brain regions; monoamine oxidase levels were elevated	Hoff 1976

Drug Category: MEPERIDINE

Human	100 mg, IM, 38-42 wk of pregnancy	general depression of fetal heart rate to sound stimulation was observed 30 min after meperidine injection	Jensen 1984
Human	1.5 mg/kg, IM during labor	fetal conc reached peak level at 1-5 hr after dose; fetal-maternal drug ratio varied between 0.35-1.5; $t_{1/2}$ averaged 3.4 hr and was not different from that in healthy control	Tomson et al. 1982
Human	50 mg, IM between 3-8 d from childbirth	meperidine appeared in milk, the conc ratio between milk and serum was greater than unity, no harmful effect in newborn	Peiker et al. 1980
Human	50 mg, IV, during labor	fetal conc of meperidine peaked 2-3 hr, that of normeperidine peaked 4 hr or later following dosing to mother	Kuhnert et al. 1979
Human	50-75 mg, IV, 4 hr before delivery	neonatal depression following meperidine & no correlation between suppression and route of administration or meperidine conc at time of delivery	Rothberg et al. 1978

Model/ Preparation	Dose/Route/Time of Exposure	Kinetic/Dynamic Effects	Reference
Human	1 mg/kg, IV, during amniotomy	decreased pH and increased pCO_2 in mother; decreased PH and base excess in fetus	Chang et al. 1976
Human	25 mg, IV infusion, during labor	no ill effects	Eliot et al. 1975
Human	50 mg, epidural analgesia, during labor	hypotension complication, decelerated fetal heart rate; neonates had lower APGAR score compared to controls	Wingate et al. 1974
Sheep	8.5-12.5 mg/kg, IV, last month of gestation	disrupted fetal sleep cycle and increased heart rate	Ruckebusch et al. 1976
Sheep	2.5 mg/kg, IV or IM, during labor	uptake of meperidine in fetal brain; peak conc of meperidine in fetal brain was 3-4 times greater from IV than IM	Szeto et al. 1980a
Sheep	3.2 mg/min, IV infusion, 111-121 d of gestation	meperidine clearance averaged 12 ml/min; ratio of meperidine clearance to inulin clearance was greater than 1, indicating tubular secretion	Szeto et al. 1980b
Sheep	2.5 mg/kg, IV, 111-121 d of gestation	meperidine $t_{1/2}$ approximated 30 hr; renal clearance varied between 2.8-16.7 ml/min; meperidine was found in amniotic and allantoic fluids	Szeto et al. 1979

Human Placenta	0.1 uCi ^{14}C-meperidine added to placenta tissue obtained 10 min after delivery	lipid-soluble analgesics crossed placenta by transcellular as well as extracellular pathways; no indication of active transport	Seeds et al. 1976
Rabbit Placenta	15 mg/hr, for 20 min, IV infusion	meperidine conc ratio between umbilical effluent and maternal plasma was 0.64; placental clearance was reduced by maternal protein binding, flow dependent at low umbilical flow rate and permeability dependent at high flow	Hamshaw-Thomas et al. 1984

Drug Category: METHADONE/METHADYL ACETATE

Human	low-dose methadone therapy	smaller head circumference, more depression of interactive behavior and state controls	Chasnoff et al. 1982
Human	methadone therapy	narcotic abstinence syndrome, smaller head circumference, elevated systolic blood pressure	Rosen & Johnson 1982
Human	50 mg/d, PO, throughout pregnancy and perinatal period	measureable but small amount of methadone in amniotic fluid & breast milk $t_{1/2}$ in neonate = 32.5 hr	Kreek 1979
Human	methadone administered to pregnant mother	cord blood level of methadone was lower than maternal serum level; conc of methadone in neonatal urine was 10-60 times that of cord blood	Harper et al. 1977

Model/ Preparation	Dose/Route/Time of Exposure	Kinetic/Dynamic Effects	Reference
Human	heroin & methadone use during pregnancy	induced chromosome damage in vivo	Abrams 1975
Human	heroin and methadone use during pregnancy	low birth rate, fetal growth retardation	Kandall 1975
Human	methadone maintenance treatment	no association of maternal dosage in last trimester of pregnancy with length of gestation, birth wt, or withdrawal syndrome; identical infant mortality rate	Newman et al. 1975
Human	methadone treatment program	increased infant mortality, decreased birth wt, increased incidence of breech presentation	Harper et al. 1974
Sheep	mother: 5 ug/kg/min fetus: 0.5 ug/kg/min IV infusion, 130-141 d of gestation	both methadone and morphine resulted in fetal arousal and suppressed quiet sleep	Umans & Szeto 1983
Sheep	methadone and morphine IV infusion, 5 hr, 130-141 d of gestation. mother: 5 ug/kg/min fetus: 0.25, or 0.5 ug/kg/min	maternal to fetal free drug concentration ratios were 7.6 for morphine and 2.9 for methadone; clearance from mother to fetus was 24.9 ml/min for morphine and 390 ml/min for methadone; fetal nonplacental clearance was 126 ml/min for morphine and 381 ml/min for methadone	Szeto et al. 1982

Sheep	5-20 mg, single dose injection to fetal circulation, 145 d of gestation	decreased carotid blood flow, decreased frequency and amplitude in EEG; electrical activity and heart rates were affected	Mann et al. 1976
Hamster	35 mg/kg, SC, during critical period of CNS organogenesis	congenital malformation of CNS, fetal anomalies	Geber & Schramm 1975
Rat	5 mg/kg/d, methadone, IP, throughout gestation and/or lactation	reduced social dominance in offspring of mothers given methadone	Thompson & Zagon 1983
Rat	0.2 or 2.0 mg/kg/d, PO, 1 mo prior to and throughout pregnancy	significant cumulation of LAAM and active metabolites in the whole fetus and fetal brain	Lichtblau et al. 1982
Rat	10 mg/kg/d, methadone PO, 5th d of gestation to term	decreased brain levels of monoamine and metabolites; methadone-exposed rats exhibited more avoidance escapes and intertrial shuttles	Rech et al. 1980
Rat	0, 4, 16 mg/kg/d, SC, 8th d of gestation to term	low body wt, high mortality, depressed open-field activity, deficits in behavioral development	Freeman 1980
Rat	0.5-2.0 mg/kg/d, PO, LAAM, chronic dosing	cumulative behavioral toxicity	Lichtblau et al. 1980
Rat	5 mg/kg/d, methadone, IP, 5 d before breeding & throughout gestation and lactation	abnormally greater wt gain during the postweaning period	McLaughlin & Zagon 1980

Model/ Preparation	Dose/Route/Time of Exposure	Kinetic/Dynamic Effects	Reference
Rat	5 mg/kg/d, methadone, SC, 14-19 d of gestation	decreased fetal testosterone and androstenedione level	Singh et al. 1980
Rat	14 mg/kg/d, methadone PO, ad lib, throughout gestation	long-lasting growth retardation and less emotionality in open-field trials	Grove et al. 1979
Rat	1-5 mg/kg, methadone, SC, bid, last trimester of pregnancy	reduction of body and brain growth	Ford & Rhines 1979
Rat	5 mg/kg, methadone, IP, during gestation and/or lactation	lower body wt, shorter crown to rump length & tail length, & smaller diameter; detrimental effect on pre-weaning organ and body development	McLaughlin et al. 1978
Rat	5 mg/kg/d, methadone, IP, during gestation & lactation	reduction of maternal wt, lower cerebellar wt & smaller width of the offspring, retarded growth and brain development of young rats	Zagon & McLaughlin 1977
Rat	2.0-8.0 mg/kg/d, methadone, IM or SC, 15-21 d of gestation	localization of methadone in fetal rat eye	Pertschuck et al. 1977
Rat	5 mg/kg/d, methadone, initially increased to 10, 15, & 20 mg/kg/d, PO, 8-22 d of gestation	blood levels were dose related; reduced maternal wt, increased mortality for the mother & the young	Hutchings et al. 1976

Rat	5-20 mg/kg/d, methadone, SC, 30 d before breeding & during pregnancy	chronic fetal methadone intoxication; increased neonatal death rate, but no evidence of development difficulty to 21 days of age	McDonald et al. 1975
Rat	25 mg/kg/d, methadone, oral gavage throughout gestation	fetal growth retardation, possible positional malformation	Chandler et al. 1975
Rat	2.5, 5.0, 7.5 mg/kg/d, methadone, IP, 1 wk before breeding	increased infant mortality, increased percentage of stillborn pups, retardation of growth, obvious dose-response relationship at low dose	Buchenauer et al. 1974
Mouse	5-28 mg/kg/d, methadone, SC, 6-15 d of gestation	reduced maternal wt gain and food consumption, increased resorptions, and decreased survival rate; adverse effects on growth development	Bui et al. 1983
Mouse	0.8, 5 mg/kg, ^3H-1-methadone, IP, 15-17 d of gestation	T_{max}=15 min in whole fetus, fetal brain,& liver; fetal brain conc were higher than maternal brain conc after 15 min	Shah et al. 1976
Drug Category: MORPHINE/HEROIN			
Human	4-6 mg, morphine, epidural injection in labor	newborn had morphine-induced respiratory depression; morphine was ineffective as an obstetric analgesic	Carlsson et al. 1981
Human	pregnant heroin addicts	elevation of chromosomal breakage, mitosis depression, chromosomal abberation	Van Blerk et al. 1980

Model/ Preparation	Dose/Route/Time of Exposure	Kinetic/Dynamic Effects	Reference
Human	narcotic (heroin and methadone) dependent women	increased pre- & post-natal growth deficiency, vascular changes, & hypoxic episodes	Finnegan 1979a
Human	pregnant drug abusers & narcotic (heroin & methadone) dependent women	mentally & neurologically deficient infants, high morbidity & mortality among newborn infants	Finnegan 1979b
Human	0.1 mg/kg, morphine or heroin, IV, in amniotomy examination	decreased PH & increased pCO_2 in mother; decreased pH & base excess in the fetus	Chang et al. 1976
Human	heroin addicts	withdrawal symptoms in infants, small body size & circumference, intrauterine growth retardation	Vargas et al. 1975
Sheep	5 mg, morphine, epidural injection, during labor	no adverse effect in mother or fetus	Craft et al. 1982
Sheep	0.66 mg/kg, morphine injection, to ewe's flank near term	altered fetal glucose & homeostasis, decreased permeability of the placenta to glucose	Raye et al. 1980
Rabbit	2.5-10 mg/kg, morphine, every 6 hr, SC, from early pregnancy till delivery	fetus weighed significantly less than controls; morphine did not accelerate fetal lung development	Roloff et al. 1975

Rat	2.5 mg/kg, morphine, IV bolus, or 23.3 ug/min/kg for 30 min, then 3.5 ug/min/kg for 30 min, 18-20 d of gestation	fetal morphine conc was 1.5 times higher than that of maternal plasma; fetal brain conc was 4 times higher than that maternal plasma	Grabrielsson & Paalzow 1983
Rat	20 mg/kg/d morphine, IV, d 12 till end of gestation	fetus showed morphine-induced depression & later developed tolerence to depressant effect <u>in utero</u>	Kirby & Holtzmann 1982
Rat	10 mg/kg, morphine, 5 mg/kg, naloxone, IP, before & during pregnancy	altered regional development of ^{3}H-methionine binding sites in the brains of offspring; affected the development of opiate receptors in brain	Tsang & Ng 1980
Rat	10 mg/kg, morphine, SC, during gestation	an enhanced prostaglandin-like activity in the homogenate of rat placenta	Scoto et al. 1979
Rat	5 mg/kg/hr for 4 hr, morphine, IV infusion, 21-22 d of gestation	caused a derangement of cerebral protein synthesis, possibly by interfering with the availability of m-RNA	Steele & Johannesson 1975a
Rat	5 mg/kg/hr for 4 hr, morphine, IV infusion, near term	inhibitory effect on transcription in fetal brain resulting from intranuclear accumulation of morphine	Steele & Johannesson 1975b
Mouse	0.12-12 mg, morphine SC; 0.068-6.5 mg/min, IV infusion; 7-10 d of pregnancy	fetal wt reduction, skeletal & soft tissue abnormalities	Ciociola & Gautieri 1983

Model/ Preparation	Dose/Route/Time of Exposure	Kinetic/Dynamic Effects	Reference
Human placenta/ Rat brain protein	1 pmole of ^{3}H-etorphine incubated with placenta mix and 0.8 mg brain protein at 37°C, 1/2 hr	human placenta exhibited lower affinity for opioid peptide than did rat brain opiate receptor	Valette et al. 1980
Human placenta	0.4-1.0 mole, morphine incubated with acetyl-choline, 37°C, 2 hr	morphine reduced ^{3}H-acetylcholine uptake	Welsch 1976
Monkey/ liver homogenate	7.25-144 umole, ethyl-morphine incubated in fetal homogenate, 12-16 wk of gestation	N-demethylation of fetal liver was 1/10 of maternal liver & adult liver	Dvorchik et al. 1974
Drug Category: NICOTINE			
Human	pregnant female smokers	atropic and hypovascular changes in placental villi, impairment of utero-placental circulation, retarded fetal growth	Mochizuki et al. 1984
Human	nursing female mokers	milk-serum conc ratio 2.92; $t_{1/2}$ of nicotine in milk slightly exceeded that in serum	Luck & Nau 1984
Human	female smokers in 2nd or 3rd trimester	fetal hypoxia, elevated levels of epinephrine, norepinephrine, and DOPEG in amniotic fluid	Divers et al. 1981

Human	pregnant female smokers	infants with low birth wt, congenital anomalies, or who died	Weathersbee & Lodge 1979
Human	habitual smoking during last trimester	increase of apnea and periodic breathing movement	Gennser et al. 1975
Human	pregnant female smokers	smaller baby, greater incidence of premature baby abortion & stillbirth	Garrett 1975
Monkey	100 ug/kg/min, 20 min, IV infusion, near term	decreased uterine blood flow, fetal acidosis & hypoxia	Suzuki et al. 1981
Monkey	1 mg/kg as single injection or infused over 20 min, 107-150 d of gestation	disappearance of nicotine from fetal circulation was slower than maternal circulation; high conc in adrenal glands, heart, kidneys, stomach wall, and spleen of fetus	Suzuki et al. 1974
Sheep	15 mg/10 min, IV infusion, 97-117 d of gestation	increased maternal arterial pH & blood pressure, increased maternal and fetal heart rates, decreased fetal arterial PCO_2 & uterine blood flow	Ayromlooi et al. 1981
Sheep	0.14-0.25 mg/kg, IV or IA, 110-120 d of gestation	decreased fetal PO_2, maternal blood flow, & fetal breathing movement; fetal hypoxemia	Manning et al. 1978
Rat	2.46 mg/d in drinking water (120 mg/l) throughout pregnancy	less maternal wt gain, higher fetal body fat, higher maternal lipolysis rate	Williams & Kanagasabai 1984

Model/ Preparation	Dose/Route/Time of Exposure	Kinetic/Dynamic Effects	Reference
Rat	1.5-3.0 mg/d, SC, 1 wk prior to mating & continued till parturation	no difference in wt gain of mother and birth wt of offspring; neurological effect on offspring, prolonged learning time	Peters & Ngan 1982
Rat	15-90 mg/30 cigarette inhalation, bid, throughout gestation	reduced maternal wt, reduced wt & length of fetus, resorption, and stillbirth	Reznik & Marquard 1980
Rat	5 mg/kg, SC, d 9 of gestation	no significant adverse effects in embryonic development and fetal viability	Lindenschmidt & Persaud 1980
Rat	0.2 mg, SC, 1-8 d of gestation	prolonged gestation period, decreased fetal number & wt	Biswas et al. 1977
Rat	6.03 mg/kg/d, PO, 0-20 d of pregnancy; 1 mg/kg, IP, single dose d 20 of pregnancy	no difference in fetal level of triglyceride, phospholipid, and cholesterol compared with control group	Mosier et al. 1974
Mouse	5.7-28.6 mg/d in drinking water (100 mg/l), 2 wk before breeding & throughout gestation	fetus weighed 12% less than control, decreased placental wt, decreased placental amino acid transport	Rowell & Clark 1982

Drug Category: PHENCYCLIDINE

Human	PCP daily, prior to and during pregnancy	sudden outbursts of agitation, rapid changes in level of consciousness, increased lability of states, and poor consolability	Chasnoff et al. 1983
Human	case study of PCP abusers	presence of PCP in breast milk and amniotic fluid	Kaufman et al. 1983
Human	PCP during first 6 wk of pregnancy	cerebellar malformation	Michaud et al. 1982
Human	irregular consumption of PCP prior to and during pregnancy	Neonates showed jitteriness, hyper-tonicity, vomiting,diarrhea, microcephaly	Strauss et al. 1981
Human	PCP abuse during pregnancy	abnormal neonatal behavior, dysmorphology, spasticity	Golden et al. 1980
Pig	2 mg/kg, IM, single dose before general anesthesia for delivery	PCP in piglet plasma 10 times higher than that in maternal sow plasma, $t_{1/2}$=6 hr in piglet, $t_{1/2}$=2 hr in adult sow	Cummings et al. 1979
Pig	0.5 g, IM, before general anesthesia for delivery	PCP in piglet plasma 10 times higher than maternal plasma, $t_{1/2}$=10-12 hr in piglet, $t_{1/2}$=2-4 hr in mother	Cooper et al. 1977
Rat	10-40 mg/kg/d, IP, 15-20 d of gestation	morphological & behavioral alterations	Jordan et al. 1979

Model/ Preparation	Dose/Route/Time of Exposure	Kinetic/Dynamic Effects	Reference
Mouse	5, 10, 20 mg/kg/d, PO, 5 d prior to mating & throughout gestation	delayed disappearance of cross extensive reflex, delayed appearance of reflexes, decreased growth rate	Nicholas & Schreiber 1983
Mouse	60–120 mg/kg/d, PO, 6–15 d of gestation	malformed fetuses at 120 mg/kg/d, but not teratogenic	Marks et al. 1980
Human Placenta	0.5 mM PCP incubated with 0.02–0.1 mg microsomal protein for 20 min, pH=8.8, T=37°C	placenta was demonstrated to be an active site of PCP biotransformation	Rayburn et al. 1984

Keys: bid=twice daily; conc=concentration; d=day; gr=group; hr=hour; IA=intraarterial; IM=intramuscular; IP=intraperitoneal; IV=intravenous; min=minute; mo=month; PO=per os; qd=once daily; SC=subcutaneous; wk=week; wt=weight

REFERENCES

Abel, E.L. Behavioral teratology of marijuana extract in rats. Neurobehav Toxicol 1:285-287, 1979.

Abel, E.L. Prenatal exposure to cannabis: A critical review of effects on growth, development and behavior. Behav Neural Biol 29:137-156, 1980.

Abel, E.L. Effects of delta-9-tetrahydrocannabinol on pregnancy and offspring in rats. Neurobehav Toxicol Teratol 6:29-32, 1984.

Abel, E.L.; Bush, R.; Dintcheff, B.A.; and Ernst, C.A. Critical periods for marijuana-induced intrauterine growth retardation in the rat. Neurobehav Toxicol Teratol 3:351-354, 1981.

Abrams, C.A. Cytogenetic risks to the offspring of pregnant addicts. Addict Dis 2:63-77, 1975.

Adams, J.; Buelke-Sam, J.; Kimmel, C.A.; and LaBorde, J.B. Behavioral alterations in rats prenatally exposed to low doses of d-amphetamine. Neurobehav Toxicol Teratol 4:63-70, 1982.

Apple, D.J., and Bennett, T.O. Multiple systemic and ocular malformations associated with maternal LSD usage. Arch Ophthalmol 92:301-303, 1974.

Ayromlooi, J.; Desiderio, D.; and Tobias, M. Effect of nicotine sulfate on the hemodynamics and acid base balance of chronically instrumented pregnant sheep. Dev Pharmacol Ther 3:205-213, 1981.

Back, D.J., and Singh, J.K.G. LSD: The distribution of [^{3}H]LSD in the reproductive system of the male rat and placental transfer in the female rat. Experientia 33:501-502, 1977.

Banerjie, B.N.; Galbreath, C.; and Sofia, R.D. Teratologic evaluation of synthetic delta-9-tetrahydrocannabinoid in rats. Teratology 11:99-101, 1975.

Bigl, V.; Dalitz, E.; Kunert, E.; Biesold, D.; and Leonard, B.E. The effect of d-amphetamine and amitriptyline administered to pregnant rats on the locomotor activity and neurotransmitters of the offspring. Psychopharmacology 77:371-375, 1982.

Billing, L.; Eriksson, M.; Larsson, G.; and Zetterstrom, R. Amphetamine addiction and pregnancy. III. One year follow-up of the children. Psychosocial and pediatric aspects. Acta Paediatr Scand 69:675-680, 1980.

Biswas, N.M.; Paul, B.; and Sarkar, D. Role of phentolamine on the length of pregnancy and fetal development in nicotine-treated pregnant rats. Endokrinologie 69:359-360, 1977.

Blackard, C., and Tennes, K. Human placental transfer of cannabinoids. N Engl J Med 311:797, 1984.

Bromley, B.L.; Rabii, J.; Gorden, J.H.; and Zimmerman, E. Delta-9-tetrahydrocannabinol inhibition of suckling-induced prolactin release in the lactating rat. Endocr Res Commun 5:271-278, 1978.

Buchenauer, D.; Turnbow, M.; and Peters, M.A. Effect of chronic methadone administration on pregnant rats and their offspring. J Pharmacol Exp Ther 189:66-71, 1974.

Bui, Q.Q.; Sperling, F.; and West, W.L. Developmental toxic effect after subcutaneous injections of methadone in Charles River CD-1 mice. Drug Chem Toxicol 6:41-70, 1983.

Carlsson, C.; Nybell-Lindahl, G.; Ingemarsson, I.; Westgren, M.; and Paalzow, L. Maternal and fetal concentrations of morphine after epidural administration during labor. Am J Obstet Gynecol 139:20-21, 1981.

Chan, C.C.; Fishman, M.; and Egbert, P.R. Multiple ocular anomalies associated with maternal LSD ingestion. Arch Ophthalmol 96:282-284, 1978.
Chandler, J.M.; Robie, P.W.; Schoolar, J.C.; and Desmond, M.M. The effects of methadone on maternal-fetal interactions in the rat. J Pharmacol Exp Ther 192:549-554, 1975.
Chang, A.; Wood, C.; Humphrey, M.; Gilbert, M.; and Wagstaff, C. The effects of narcotics on fetal acid base status. Br J Obstet Gynaecol 83:56-61, 1976.
Chasnoff, I.J.; Hatcher, R.; and Burns, W.J. Polydrug- and methadone-addicted newborns: A continuum of impairment? Pediatrics 70:210-213, 1982.
Chasnoff, I.J.; Burns, W.J.; Hatcher, R.P.; and Burns, K.A. Phencyclidine: Effects on the fetus and neonate. Dev Pharmacol Ther 6:404-408, 1983.
Ciociola, A.A., and Gautieri, R.F. Evaluation of the teratogenicity of morphine sulfate administered via a miniature implantable pump. J Pharm Sci 72:742-745, 1983.
Cooper, E.J.; Cummings, A.J.; and Jones, H. The placental transfer of phencyclidine in the pig: Plasma levels in the sow and its piglets. J Physiol (Lond) 267:11-18, 1977.
Cotterill, R.W.; Penney, L.L.; Vaughn, D.L.; Reimann, B.E.; and Rauls, D.O. Acute cardiovascular effects of delta-9-tetrahydrocannabinol in pregnant anesthetized sheep. Biol Res Pregnancy Perinatol 5:1-5, 1984.
Coyle, I.; Wayner, M.J.; and Singer, G. Behavioral teratogenesis: A critical evaluation. Pharmacol Biochem Behav 4:191-200, 1976.
Craft, J.B., Jr.; Bolan, J.C.; Coaldrake, L.A.; Mondino, M.; Mazel, P.; Gilman, R.M.; Shokes, L.K.; and Woolf, W.A. The maternal and fetal cardiovascular effects of epidural morphine in the sheep model. Am J Obstet Gynecol 142:835-839, 1982.
Cummings, A.J.; Jones, H.M.; and Cooper, J.E. Transplacental disposition of phencyclidine in the pig. Xenobiotica 9:447-452, 1979.
Dalterio, S.L. Perinatal or adult exposure to cannabinoids alters male reproductive functions in mice. Pharmacol Biochem Behav 12:145-153, 1980.
Dalterio, S., and Bartke, A. Fetal testosterone in mice: Effect of gestational age and cannabinoid exposure. J Endocrinol 91:509-514, 1981.
Dalterio, S.; Steger, R.; Mayfield, D.; and Bartke, A. Early cannabinoid exposure influences neuroendocrine and reproductive functions in male mice: I. Prenatal exposure. Pharmacol Biochem Behav 20:107-113, 1984a.
Dalterio, S.; Steger, R.; Mayfield, D.; and Bartke, A. Early cannabinoid exposure influences neuroendocrine and reproductive functions in mice: II. Postnatal effects. Pharmacol Biochem Behav 20:115-123, 1984b.
Dishotsky, N.I.; Loughman, W.D.; Magar, R.E.; and Lipscomb, W.R. LSD and genetic damage. Science 172:431-440, 1971.
Divers, W.A., Jr.; Wilkes, M.M.; Babaknia, A.; and Yen, S.S. Maternal smoking and elevation of catecholamines and metabolites in the amniotic fluid. Am J Obstet Gynecol 141:625-628, 1981.
Dvorchik, B.H.; Stenger, B.G.; and Quattropani, S.L. Fetal hepatic drug metabolism in the nonhuman primate, Macaca arctoides. Drug Metab Dispos 74:539-544, 1974.

Eliot, B.W.; Hill, J.G.; Cole, A.P.; and Hailey, D.M. Continuous pethidine/diazepam infusion during labour and its effects on the newborn. Br J Obstet Gynaecol 82:126-131, 1975.
Eriksson, M.; Larsson, G.; and Zetterstrom, R. Amphetamine addiction and pregnancy. II. Pregnancy, delivery and the neonatal period. Socio-medical aspects. Acta Obstet Gynecol Scand 60:253-259, 1981
Fantel, A.G., and Macphail, B.J. The teratogenicity of cocaine. Teratology 26:17-19, 1982.
Fernandez, J.; Brennan, T.; Masterson, J.; and Power, M. Cytogenetic studies in the offspring of LSD users. Br J Psychiatry 124:296-298, 1974.
Finnegan, L.P. In utero opiate dependence and sudden infant death syndrome. Clin Perinatol 6:163-180, 1979a.
Finnegan, L.P. Pathophysiological and behavioral effects of the transplacental transfer of narcotic drugs to the fetuses and neonates of narcotic-dependent mothers. Bull Narc 31:1-58, 1979b.
Fleischman, R.W.; Hayden, D.W.; Rosenkrantz, H.; and Braude, M.C. Teratologic evaluation of delta-9-tetrahydrocannabinol in mice, including a review of the literature. Teratology 12:47-50, 1975.
Fleischman, R.W.; Naqui, R.H.; Rosenkrantz, H.; and Hayden, D.W. The embryotoxic effects of cannabinoids in rats and mice. J Environ Pathol Toxicol 4:471-482, 1980.
Ford, D.H., and Rhines, R.K. Prenatal exposure to methadone HCl in relationship to body and brain growth in the rat. Acta Neurol Scand 59:248-262, 1979.
Freeman, R.R. Methadone exposure in utero: Effects on open-field activity in weaning rats. Int J Neurosci 11:295-300, 1980.
Fried, P.A. Marijuana use by pregnant women: Neurobehavioral effects in neonates. Drug Alcohol Depend 6:414-424, 1980
Fried, P.A., and Charlebois, A.T. Effects upon rat offspring following cannabis inhalation before and/or after mating. Can J Psychol 33:125-132, 1979.
Frischknecht, H.R.; Sieber, B.; and Waser, P.G. The feeding of hashish to lactating mice: Effects on the development of suckings. Gen Pharmacol 11:469-472, 1980.
Frischknecht, H.R.; Sieber, B.; and Waser, P.G. Effects of multiple, chron-
ic and early hashish exposure on mating behavior, nest-building and gestation in mice. Comp Biochem Physiol 72:363-368, 1982.
Gabrielsson, J.L., and Paalzow, L.K. A physiological pharmacokinetic model for morphine disposition in the pregnant rat. J Pharmacokinet Biopharm 11:147-163, 1983.
Garrett, R.J. Nicotine and placental iron transport. Experientia 31:486-488, 1975.
Geber, W.F., and Schramm, L.C. Congenital malformations of the central nervous system produced by narcotic analgesics in the hamster. Am J Obstet Gynecol 123:705-713, 1975.
Gennser, G.; Marsal, K.; and Brantmark, B. Maternal smoking and fetal breathing movements. Am J Obstet Gynecol 123:861-867, 1975.
Golden, N.L.; Sokol, R.J.; and Rubin, I.L. Angel dust: Possible effects on the fetus. Pediatrics 65:18-20, 1980.
Golub, M.S.; Sassenrath, E.N.; and Chapman, L.F. Mother-infant interaction in rhesus monkeys treated clinically with delta-9-tetrahydrocannabinol. Child Dev 52:389-392, 1981.

Golub, M.S.; Sassenrath, E.N.; and Chapman, L.F. An analysis of altered attention in monkeys exposed to delta-9-tetrahydrocannabinol during development. Neurobehav Toxicol Teratol 4:469-472, 1982.

Greenland, S.; Staisch, K.J.; Brown, N.; and Gross, S.J. The effects of marijuana use during pregnancy. I. A preliminary epidemiologic study. Am J Obstet Gynecol 143:408-413, 1982.

Grove, L.V.; Etkin, M.K.; and Rosecrans, J.A. Behavioral effects of fetal and neonatal exposure to methadone in the rat. Neurobehav Toxicol 1:87-95, 1979.

Hamshaw-Thomas, A.; Rogerson, N.; and Reynolds, F. Transfer of bupivacaine, lignocaine and pethidine across the rabbit placenta: Influence of maternal protein binding and fetal flow. Placenta 5:61-70, 1984.

Harper, R.G.; Solish, G.I.; Purow, H.M.; Sang, E.; and Panepinto, W.C. The effect of a methadone treatment program upon pregnant heroin addicts and their newborn infants. Pediatrics 54:300-305, 1974.

Harper, R.G.; Solish, G.; Feingold, E.; Gersten-Woolf, N.B.; and Sokal, M.M. Maternal ingested methadone, body fluid methadone, and the neonatal withdrawal syndrome. Am J Obstet Gynecol 129:417-424, 1977.

Hatoum, N.S.; Davis, W.M; Elsohly, M.A.; and Turner, C.E. Perinatal exposure to cannabichromene and delta-9-tetrahydrocannabinol: Separate and combined effects on viability of pups and on male reproductive system at maturity. Toxicol Lett 8:141-146, 1981.

Heikkila, J.J.; Holbrook, L.; and Brown, I.R. Disaggregation of polysomes in fetal organs and maternal brain after administration of d-lysergic acid diethylamide in vivo. J Neurochem 32:1793-1799, 1979.

Hitzemann, B.A.; Hitzemann, R.J.; Brase, D.A.; and Loh, H.H. Influence of prenatal d-amphetamine administration on development and behavior of rats. Life Sci 18:605-612, 1976.

Hoff, K.M. Effects of prenatal and postnatal exposure to LSD on brain maturation. Gen Pharmacol 7:395-398, 1976.

Hutchings, D.E.; Hunt, H.F.; Towly, J.P.; Rosen, T.S.; and Gorinson, H.S. Methadone during pregnancy in the rat: Dose level effects on maternal and perinatal mortality and growth in the offspring. J Pharmacol Exp Ther 197:171-179, 1976.

Jacobson, C.B., and Berlin, C.M. Possible reproductive detriment in LSD users. JAMA 222:1367-1373, 1972.

Jensen, O.H. Fetal heart rate response to sound stimulation after pethidine injection in the mother. Acta Obstet Gynecol Scand 63:1-5, 1984.

Joneja, M.G. A study of teratological effects of intravenous, subcutaneous and intragastric administration of delta-9-tetrahydrocannabinol in mice. Toxicol Appl Pharmacol 36:151-162, 1976.

Joneja, M.G. Effects of delta-9-tetrahydrocannabinol on hamster fetuses. J Toxicol Environ Health 2:1031-1040, 1977.

Jordan, R.L.; Young, T.R.; Dinwiddie, S.H.; and Harry, G.L. Phencyclidine-induced morphological and behavioral alterations in the neonatal rat. Pharmacol Biochem Behav 11(Supp):39-45, 1979.

Kandall, S.R.; Albin, S.; Dreyer, E.; Comstock, M.; and Lowinson, J. Differential effects of heroin and methadone on birth weights. Addict Dis 2:347-355, 1975.

Kaufman, K.R.; Petrucha, R.A.; Pitt, F.N., Jr.; and Weekes, M.E. PCP in amniotic fluid and breast milk: Case report. J Clin Psychiatry 44:269-70, 1983.

Kawash, G.F.; Young, D.L.; and Berg, S.D. Effects of administration of cannabis resin during pregnancy on emotionality and learning in rat's offspring. Percept Mot Skills 50:358-365, 1980.
Kirby, M.L., and Holtzmann, S.G. Effects of chronic opiate administration on spontaneous activity of fetal rats. Pharmacol Biochem Behav 16:263-269, 1982.
Kostellow, A.B.; Ziegler, D.; Kunar, J.; Fujimoto, G.I.; and Morrill, G.A. Effect of cannabinoids on estrous cycle, ovulation and reproduction capacity of female A/J mice. Pharmacology 21:68-75, 1980.
Kreek, M.J. Methadone disposition during the perinatal period in humans. Pharmacol Biochem Behav 11(Supp):7-13, 1979.
Kuhnert, B.R.; Kuhnert, P.M.; Tu, A.S.; and Line, D.C. Meperidine and normeperidine levels following meperidine administration during labor II. Fetus and neonate. Am J Obstet Gynecol 133:909-914, 1979.
Kulay, L., Jr.; Oliveira-Filho, R.M.; Siciliano, and S.F.; Kulay, M.N. The effect of N-2-cyano-ethylamphetamine HCl on total lipid contents of placenta and some maternal and fetal tissues of the rat. Rev Bras Pesqui Med Biol 11:325-328, 1978.
Lichtblau, L.; Burklund, K.E.; and Sparber, S.B. A method for determining cumulative behavioral toxicity after chronic oral administration of 1-alpha-acetylmethadol to female rats. Neurobehav Toxicol 2:13-19, 1980.
Lichtblau, L.; Finkle, B.S.; and Sparber, S.B. Cumulation of active metabolites of levo-alpha-acetylmethadol in the rat fetus and neonate. Life Sci 30:307-312, 1982.
Lindenschmidt, R.R., and Persaud, T.V. Effect of ethanol and nicotine in the pregnant rat. Res Commun Chem Pathol Pharmacol 27:195-198, 1980.
Long, S.Y. Does LSD induce chromosomal damage and malformations? A review of literature. Teratology 6:75-90, 1972
Luck, W., and Nau, H. Nicotine and continine concentrations in serum and milk of nursing smokers. Br J Clin Pharmacol 18:9-15, 1984.
Mahalik, M.P.; Gautieri, R.F.; and Mann, D.E., Jr. Teratogenic potential of cocaine hydrochloride in CF-1 mice. J Pharm Sci 69:703-706, 1980.
Mann, L.I.; Bhakthewathsalan, A.; Liu, M.; and Makowski, P. The effect of methadone on fetal brain function. Am J Obstet Gynecol 124:699-704, 1976.
Manning, F.; Walker, D.; and Feyerabend, C. The effect of nicotine on fetal breathing movements in conscious pregnant ewes. Obstet Gynecol 52:563-568, 1978.
Mantilla-Plata B., and Harbison, R.D. Alteration of delta-9-tetrahydrocannabinol-induced prenatal toxicity by phenobarbital and SKF-525A. In: Nahas, G.G., and Paton, S.W., eds. Marihuana: chemistry, biochemistry and cellular effects. New York: Springer, 1976. pp. 457-468.
Margolis, S., and Martin, L. Anophthalmia in an infant of parents using LSD. Ann Ophthalmol 12:1378-1381, 1980.
Marks, T.A.; Worthy, W.C.; and Staples, R.E. Teratogenic potential of phencyclidine in mouse. Teratology 21:541-546, 1980.
Martin, B.R.; Dewey, W.L.; Harris, L.S.; and Beckner, J.S. ^{3}H-Delta-9-tetrahydrocannabinol distribution in pregnant dogs and their fetuses. Res Commun Chem Pathol Pharmacol 17:457-470, 1977.

Martin, J.C. Effects on offspring of chronic maternal methamphetamine exposure. Dev Psychobiol 8:397-404, 1975.

Martin, J.C., and Martin, D.C. Voluntary activity in the aging rat as a function of maternal drug exposure. Neurobehav Toxicol Teratol 3:261-264, 1981.

Martin, J.C.; Martin, D.C.; Radow, B.; and Sigman, G. Growth, development and activity in rat offspring following maternal drug exposure. Exp Aging Res 2:235-251, 1976.

Martin, J.C.; Martin, D.D.; Radow, B.; and Day H.E. Life span and pathology in offspring following nicotine and methamphetamine exposure. Exp Aging Res 5:509-522, 1979.

McDonald, L.K.; Maddux, J.F.; and Blum, K. Fetal consequences of chronic methadone administration to pregnant rats: Methodological problems. Curr Ther Res 17:308-317, 1975.

McLaughlin, P.J., and Zagon, I.S. Body and organ development of young rats maternally exposed to methadone. Biol Neonate 38:185-196, 1980.

McLaughlin, P.J.; Zagon, I.S.; and White, W.J. Perinatal methadone exposure in rats. Effects on body and organ development. Biol Neonate 34:48-54, 1978.

Michaud, J.; Mizraki, E.M.; and Urich, H. Agenesis of the vermis with fusion of the cerebellar hemispheres, septo-optic dysplasia and associated anomalies: Report of a case. Acta Neuropathol (Berl) 56:161-166, 1982.

Middaugh, L.D.; Blackwell, L.A.; Santos, C.A.; and Zemp, J.W. Effects of d-amphetamine sulfate given to pregnant mice on activity and on catecholamines in the brains of offspring. Dev Psychobiol 7:429-438, 1974.

Milkovich, L., and van den Berg, B.J. Effects of antenatal exposure to anorectic drugs. Am J Obstet Gynecol 129:637-642, 1977.

Mochizuki, M.; Maruo, T.; Masuko, K.; and Ohtsu, T. Effects of smoking on feto-placental-maternal system during pregnancy. Am J Obstet Gynecol 149:413-420, 1984.

Monder, H. Effects of prenatal amphetamine exposure on the development of behavior in rats. Psychopharmacology 75:75-78, 1981.

Mosier, H.D., Jr; Capodanno, C.C.; Li, I.O.; Magruder, C.S.; and Jansons, R.A. Resistance of rat fetuses to nicotine-induced lipolysis. Teratology 9:239-245, 1974.

Naeye, R.L. Maternal use of dextroamphetamine and growth of the fetus. Pharmacology 26:117-120, 1983.

Nasello, A.G., and Ramirez, O.A. Brain catecholamines metabolism in offspring of amphetamine treated rats. Pharmacol Biochem Behav 9:17-20, 1978a.

Nasello, A.G., and Ramirez, O.A. Open-field and Lashley III maze behaviour of the offspring of ampehtamine-treated rats. Psychopharmacology 58:171-173, 1978b

Nasello, A.G.; Astrada, C.A.; and Ramirez, O.A. Effects on the acquisition of conditioned avoidance responses and seizure threshold in the offspring of amphetamine treated gravid rats. Psychopharmacologia 40:25-31, 1974.

Newman, R.G.; Bashkow, S.; and Calko, D. Results of 313 consecutive live births of infants delivered to patients in the New York City Methadone Maintenance Treatment Program. Am J Obstet Gynecol 121:233-237, 1975.

Nicholas, J.M., and Schreiber, E.C. Phencyclidine exposure and the developing mouse: Behavioral teratological implications. Teratology 28:319-326, 1983.

Parker, W.A. Effects of pregnancy on pharmacokinetics. In: Benet, L.Z.; Massoud, N.; and Gambertoglio, J.G., eds. Pharmacokinetic Basis for Drug Treatment. New York: Raven Press, 1984. pp.249-268.

Peiker, G.; Muller, B.; Ihn, W.; and Noschel, H. Excretion of pethidine in mother's milk. Zentralbl Gynakol 102:537-541, 1980.

Perez-Reyes, M. Presence of delta-9-tetrahydrocannabinol in human milk. N Engl J Med 307:819-820, 1982.

Pertschuk, L.P.; Ford, D.H.; and Rainford, E.A. Localization of methadone in fetal rat eye by the immunofluorescence technic. Exp Eye Res 24:547-552, 1977.

Peters, M.A. Development of a "blood-brain barrier" to methadone in the newborn rat. J Pharmacol Exp Ther 192:513-520, 1975.

Peters, M.A., and Ngan, L.L. The effects of totigestational exposure to nicotine on pre- and post-natal development in the rat. Arch Int Pharmacodyn Ther 257:155-167, 1982.

Raine, J.M.; Wing, D.R.; and Paton, W.D. The effects of delta-9-tetrahydrocannabinol on mammary gland growth, enzyme activity and plasma prolactin levels in the mouse. Eur J Pharmacol 51:11-17, 1978.

Ramirez, O.A.; Carrer, H.F.; and Nasello, A.G. Prenatal amphetamine exposure: Ovulation, sexual behavior and hypothalamic monoamine content in rats. Pharmacol Biochem Behav 11:605-609, 1979.

Ramirez, O.A.; Keller, E.A.; and Orsingher, O.A. Prenatal amphetamine reduces alpha but not beta adrenergic receptor binding in brain of adult rats. Life Sci 32:1835-1838, 1983

Rayburn, W.F.; Holsztynska, E.F.; and Domino, E.F. Phencyclidine: Biotransformation by the human placenta. Am J Obstet Gynecol 148:111-112, 1984.

Raye, J.R.; Dubin, J.W.; and Blechner, J.N. Alterations in fetal metabolism subsequent to maternal morphine administration. Am J Obstet Gynecol 137:505-508, 1980.

Rech, R.H.; Lomuscio, G.; and Algeri, S. Methadone exposure in utero: Effects on brain biogenic amines and behavior. Neurobehav Toxicol 2:75-78, 1980.

Reznik, G., and Marquard, G. Effect of cigarette smoke inhalation during pregnancy in Sprague-Dawley rats. J Environ Pathol Toxicol 4:141-152, 1980.

Robinson, J.T.; Chitham, R.G.; Greenwood, R.M.; and Taylor, J.W. Chromosome aberrations and LSD. A controlled study in 50 psychiatric patients. Br J Psychiatry 125:238-244, 1974.

Roloff, D.W.; Howatt, W.F.; Kanto, W.P., Jr.; and Borker, R.C., Jr. Morphine administration to pregnant rabbits: Effect on fetal growth and lung development. Addict Dis 2:369-379, 1975.

Rosen, T.S., and Johnson, H.L. Children of methadone-maintained mothers: Follow-up to 18 months of age. J Pediatr 101:192-196, 1982.

Rosenkrantz, H., and Esber, H.J. Cannabinoid-induced hormone changes in monkeys and rats. J Toxicol Environ Health 6:297-313, 1980.

Rothberg, R.M.; Rieger, C.H..; Hill, J.H.; Danielson, J.; and Matadial L. Cord and maternal serum meperidine concentrations and clinical status of the infant. Biol Neonate 33:80-89, 1978.

Rowell, P.P., and Clark, M.J. The effect of chronic oral nicotine administration on fetal weight and placental amino acid accumulation in mice. Toxicol Appl Pharmacol 66:30-38, 1982.

Ruckebusch, Y.; Gaujoux, M.; and Eghbali, B. Placental transfer of central nervous system depressants in sheep. Eur J Pharmacol 37:193-196, 1976.

Sastry, B.V.; Olubadewo, J.O.; and Boehm, F.H. Effects of nicotine and cocaine on the release of acetylcholine from isolated human placental villi. Arch Int Pharmacodyn Ther 229:23-26, 1977.

Satinder, K.P., and Sterling, J.W. Differential effects of pre- and/or post-natal d-amphetamine on avoidance response in genetically selected lines of rats. Neurobehav Toxicol Teratol 5:315-320, 1983.

Scoto, G.M.; Spadaro, C.; Spampinato, S.,; Nossan, N.; Arrigo-Reina, R.; and Ferri, S. Prostaglandins in rat placenta following acute and chronic administration of morphine. Arch Toxicol Suppl 2:375-380, 1979.

Seeds, A.E.; Stolee, A.; and Eichhorst, B.C. Permeability of human chorion laeve to diazepam and meperidine. Obstet Gynecol 47:28-30, 1976.

Seliger, D.L. Prenatal maternal d-amphetamine effects on emotionality and audiogenic seizure susceptibility of rat offspring. Dev Psychobiol 8:261-268, 1975.

Shah, N.S., and Yates J.D. Placental transfer and tissue distribution of dextro-amphetamine in the mouse. Arch Int Pharmacodyn Ther 233:200-208, 1978.

Shah, N.S.; Donald, A.G.; Bertolatus, J.A.; and Hixson, B. Tissue distribution of levo-methadone in nonpregnant and pregnant female and male mice: Effect of SKF 525-A-1,2. J Pharmacol Exp Ther 199:103-116, 1976.

Shah, N.S.; May, D.A.; and Yates, J.D. Disposition of levo-^{3}H-cocaine in pregnant and nonpregnant mice. Toxicol Appl Pharmacol 53:279-284, 1980

Singh, H.H.; Purohit, V.; and Ahluewalia, B.S. Effect of methadone treatment during pregnancy on the fetal testes and hypothalamus in rats. Biol Reprod 22:480-485, 1980.

Slone, D.; Shapiro, S.; and Mitchell, A.A. Strategies for studying the effects of the antenatal chemical environment on the fetus. In: Schwartz, R.H., and Yaffe, S.T., eds. Drug and Chemical Risks to the Fetus and Newborn. New York: Alan R. Liss, Inc., 1980. pp.1-8.

Sofia, R.D.; Strasbough, J.E.; and Banerjee, B.N. Teratologic evaluation of synthetic delta-9-tetrahydrocannabinol in rabbits. Teratology 19:361-366, 1979.

Steele, W.J., and Johannesson, T. Effects of morphine infusion in maternal rats at near-term on ribosome size distribution in foetal and maternal rat brain. Acta Pharmacol Toxicol 36:236-242, 1975a.

Steele, W.J., and Johannesson, T. Distribution of ^{14}C-morphine and macromolecules in the brain and liver and their nuclei in pregnant rats and their foetuses after infusion of morphine into pregnant rats at nearterm. Acta Pharmacol Toxicol 37:265-273, 1975b.

Strauss, A.A.; Modaniou; H.D.; and Bosu, S.K. Neonatal manifestations of maternal phencyclidine (PCP) abuse. Pediatrics 68:550-552, 1981.

Suzuki, K.; Horiguchi, T.; Comas-Urrutia, A.C.; Mueller-Heubach, E.; Morishima, H.O., and Adamsons, K. Placental transfer and distribution of nicotine in the pregnant rhesus monkey. Am J Obstet Gynecol 119:253-262, 1974.

Suzuki, K.; Minei, L.J.; and Johnson, E.E. Effect of nicotine upon uterine blood flow in the pregnant rhesus monkey. Teratology 23:259-271, 1981.

Szeto, H.H.; Kaiko, R.F.; Clapp, J.F.; Larrow, R.W.; Mann, L.I.; and Inturrisi, C.E. Urinary excretion of meperidine by the fetal lamb. J Pharmacol Exp Ther 209:244-248, 1979.

Szeto, H.H.; Clapp, J.F.; Abrams, R.; Inturrisi, C.E.; Kaiko, R.F.; Larrow, R.W.; and Mann, L.I. Brain uptake of meperidine in the fetal lamb. Am J Obstet Gynecol 138:528-533, 1980a.

Szeto, H.H,; Clapp, J.F.; Larrow, R.W.; Inturrisi, C.E.; and Mann, L.I. Renal tubular secretion of meperidine by the fetal lamb. J Pharmacol Exp Ther 213:346-349, 1980b.

Szeto, H.H.; Umans, J.G.; and McFarland, J. A comparison of morphine and methadone disposition in the maternal-fetal unit. Am J Obstet Gynecol 143:700-706, 1982.

Thompson, C.I., and Zagon, I.S. Reduced social dominance in rats perinatally exposed to methadone. Neurobehav Toxicol Teratol 5:17-21, 1983.

Tomson, G.; Garle, R.I.; Thalme, B.; Nisell, H.; Nylund, L.; and Rane, A. Maternal kinetics and transplacental passage of pethidine during labour. Br J Clin Pharmacol 13:653-659, 1982.

Tsang, D., and Ng, S.C. Effect of antenatal exposure to opiates on the development of opiate receptors in rat brain. Brain Res 188:199-206, 1980.

Umans, J.G., and Szeto, H.H. Effects of opiates on fetal behavioral activity in utero. Life Sci 33 (Supp): 639-642, 1983.

Valette, A.; Reme, J.M.; Pontonnier, G.; and Cross, J. Specific binding for opiate-like drugs in the placenta. Biochem Pharmacol 29:2657-2662, 1980.

Van Blerk, G.A.; Majerus, T.C.; and Myers, R.A. Teratogenic potential of some psychopharmacologic drugs: A brief review. Int J Gynaecol Obstet 17:399-402, 1980.

Vardaris, R.M.; Weisz, D.J.; Fazel, A.; and Rawitch, A.B. Chronic administration of delta-9-tetrahydrocannabinol to pregnant rats: Studies of pup behavior and placental transfer. Pharmacol Biochem Behav 4:249-254, 1976.

Vargas, G.C.; Pildes, R.S.; Vidyasagar, D.; and Keith, L.G. Effects of maternal heroin addiction on 67 liveborn neonates. Clin Pediatr (Phila) 14:651-753, 1975.

Weathersbee, P.S., and Lodge, J.R. Alcohol, caffeine, and nicotine as factors in pregnancy. Postgrad Med 66:165-167, 170-171, 1979.

Welsch, F. Effects of drugs on the uptake of acetylcholine by human term placenta fragments. Res Commun Chem Pathol Pharmacol 15:457-468, 1976.

Williams, C.M., and Kanagasabai, T. Maternal adipose tissue response to nicotine administration in the pregnant rat: Effects on fetal body fat and cellularity. Br J Nutr 51:7-13, 1984.

Wingate, M.B.; Wingate, L.; Iffy, L.; Freundlich, J.; and Gottsegen, D. The effect of epidural analgesia upon fetal and neonatal status. Am J Obstet Gynecol 119:1101-1106, 1974.

Wright, P.L.; Smith, S.H.; Keplinger, M.L.; Calandra, J.C.; and Braude, M.C. Reproductive and teratologic studies with delta-9-tetrahydrocannabinol and crude marijuana extract. Toxicol Appl Pharmacol 38:223-235, 1976.

Zagon, I.S., and McLaughlin, P.J. Effect of chronic maternal methadone exposure on perinatal development. Biol Neonate 31:271-282, 1977.

AUTHORS

Charles C. Lee, Ph.D.
University of Houston
Texas Medical Center
1441 Moursund Ave.
Houston, Texas 77030

C. Nora Chiang, Ph.D.
Division of Preclinical Research
National Institute on Drug Abuse
5600 Fishers Lane
Rockville, Maryland 20857

National Institute on Drug Abuse

Research

monograph series

While limited supplies last, single copies of the monographs may be obtained free of charge from the National Clearinghouse for Drug Abuse Information (NCDAI). Please contact NCDAI also for information about availability of coming issues and other publications of the National Institute on Drug Abuse relevant to drug abuse research.

Additional copies may be purchased from the U.S. Government Printing Office (GPO) and/or the National Technical Information Service (NTIS) as indicated. For the most recent monographs, stock numbers and prices may not be shown because they had not been assigned when this monograph went to press. NTIS prices are for paper copy. Microfiche copies, at $4.50, are also available from NTIS. Prices from either source are subject to change.

Addresses are:

NCDAI
National Clearinghouse for Drug Abuse Information
Room 10A-43
5600 Fishers Lane
Rockville, Maryland 20857

GPO
Superintendent of Documents
U.S. Government Printing Office
Washington, D.C. 20402

NTIS
National Technical Information Service
U.S. Department of Commerce
Springfield, Virginia 22161

1 FINDINGS OF DRUG ABUSE RESEARCH. NCDAI out of stock
Vol. 1: GPO out of stock NTIS PB #272 867/AS $32.50
Vol. 2: GPO out of stock NTIS PB #272 868/AS $29.50

2 OPERATIONAL DEFINITIONS IN SOCIO-BEHAVIORAL DRUG USE RESEARCH 1975. Jack Elinson, Ph.D., and David Nurco, Ph.D., eds. NCDAI out of stock GPO out of stock NTIS PB #246 338/AS $16

3 AMINERGIC HYPOTHESES OF BEHAVIOR: REALITY OR CLICHE? Bruce J. Bernard, Ph.D., ed. NCDAI out of stock
GPO out of stock NTIS PB #246 687/AS $16

4 NARCOTIC ANTAGONISTS: THE SEARCH FOR LONG-ACTING PREPARATIONS. Robert Willette, Ph.D., ed.
GPO out of stock NTIS PB #247 096/AS $8.50

5 YOUNG MEN AND DRUGS: A NATIONWIDE SURVEY. John A. O'Donnell, Ph.D., et al. NCDAI out of stock
GPO out of stock NTIS PB #247 446/AS $16

6 EFFECTS OF LABELING THE "DRUG ABUSER": AN INQUIRY. Jay R. Williams, Ph.D. NCDAI out of stock
GPO out of stock NTIS PB #249 092/AS $8.50

7 CANNABINOID ASSAYS IN HUMANS. Robert Willette, Ph.D., ed. NCDAI out of stock
GPO Stock #017-024-01151-7 $5 NTIS PB #251 905/AS $14.50

8 Rx: 3x/WEEK LAAM - ALTERNATIVE TO METHADONE. Jack Blaine, M.D., and Pierre Renault, M.D., eds.
Not available from GPO NTIS PB #253 763/AS $14.50

9 NARCOTIC ANTAGONISTS: NALTREXONE PROGRESS REPORT. Demetrios Julius, M.D., and Pierre Renault, M.D., eds. NCDAI out of stock
GPO out of stock NTIS PB #255 833/AS $17.50

10 EPIDEMIOLOGY OF DRUG ABUSE: CURRENT ISSUES. Louise G. Richards, Ph.D., and Louise B. Blevens, eds. NCDAI out of stock
GPO out of stock NTIS PB #266 691/AS $22

11 DRUGS AND DRIVING. Robert Willette, Ph.D., ed. NCDAI out of stock
GPO Stock #017-024-00576-2 $5.50 NTIS PB #269 602/AS $16

12 PSYCHODYNAMICS OF DRUG DEPENDENCE. Jack D. Blaine, M.D., and Demetrios A. Julius, M.D., eds. NCDAI out of stock
GPO out of stock NTIS PB #276 084/AS $17.50

13 COCAINE: 1977. Robert C. Petersen, Ph.D., and Richard C. Stillman, M.D., eds. NCDAI out of stock
GPO out of stock NTIS PB #269 175/AS $19

14 MARIHUANA RESEARCH FINDINGS: 1976. Robert C. Petersen, Ph.D., ed. NCDAI out of stock
GPO out of stock NTIS PB #271 279/AS $22

15 REVIEW OF INHALANTS: EUPHORIA TO DYSFUNCTION. Charles Wm. Sharp, Ph.D., and Mary Lee Brehm, Ph.D., eds.
GPO out of stock NTIS PB #275 798/AS $28

16 THE EPIDEMIOLOGY OF HEROIN AND OTHER NARCOTICS. Joan Dunne Rittenhouse, Ph.D., ed. NCDAI out of stock
GPO out of stock NTIS PB #276 357/AS $20.50

17 RESEARCH ON SMOKING BEHAVIOR. Murray E. Jarvik, M.D., Ph.D., et al., eds. NCDAI out of stock
GPO out of stock NTIS PB #276 353/AS $29.50

18 BEHAVIORAL TOLERANCE: RESEARCH AND TREATMENT IMPLICATIONS. Norman A. Krasnegor, Ph.D., ed.
GPO out of stock NTIS PB #276 337/AS $16

19 THE INTERNATIONAL CHALLENGE OF DRUG ABUSE. Robert C. Petersen, Ph.D., ed.
GPO out of stock NTIS PB #293 807/AS $28

20 SELF-ADMINISTRATION OF ABUSED SUBSTANCES: METHODS FOR STUDY. Norman A. Krasnegor, Ph.D., ed.
GPO out of stock NTIS PB #288 471/AS $22

21 PHENCYCLIDINE (PCP) ABUSE: AN APPRAISAL. Robert C. Petersen, Ph.D., and Richard C. Stillman, M.D., eds.
GPO out of stock NTIS PB #288 472/AS $25

22 QUASAR: QUANTITATIVE STRUCTURE ACTIVITY RELATIONSHIPS OF ANALGESICS, NARCOTIC ANTAGONISTS, AND HALLUCINOGENS. Gene Barnett, Ph.D.; Milan Trsic, Ph.D.; and Robert Willette, Ph.D.; eds. NCDAI out of stock
GPO out of stock NTIS PB #292 265/AS $35.50

23 CIGARETTE SMOKING AS A DEPENDENCE PROCESS. Norman A. Krasnegor, Ph.D., ed. NCDAI out of stock
GPO Stock #017-024-00895-8 $6 NTIS PB #297 721/AS $19

24 SYNTHETIC ESTIMATES FOR SMALL AREAS: STATISTICAL WORKSHOP PAPERS AND DISCUSSION. Jos. Steinberg, ed. NCDAI out of stock
GPO out of stock NTIS PB #299 009/AS $23.50

25 BEHAVIORAL ANALYSIS AND TREATMENT OF SUBSTANCE ABUSE. Norman A. Krasnegor, Ph.D., ed.
GPO ouf of stock NTIS PB #80-112428 $22

26 THE BEHAVIORAL ASPECTS OF SMOKING. Norman A. Krasnegor, Ph.D., ed.
GPO out of stock NTIS PB #80-118755 $17.50

27 PROBLEMS OF DRUG DEPENDENCE, 1979: PROCEEDINGS OF THE 41ST ANNUAL SCIENTIFIC MEETING, THE COMMITTEE ON PROBLEMS OF DRUG DEPENDENCE, INC. L.S. Harris, Ph.D., ed. NCDAI out of stock
GPO Stock #017-024-00981-4 $9 NTIS PB #80-175482 $37

28 NARCOTIC ANTAGONISTS: NALTREXONE PHARMACOCHEMISTRY AND SUSTAINED-RELEASE PREPARATIONS. Robert Willette, Ph.D., and Gene Barnett, Ph.D., eds. NCDAI out of stock
GPO out of stock NTIS PB #81-238875 $23.50

29 DRUG ABUSE DEATHS IN NINE CITIES: A SURVEY REPORT. Louis A. Gottschalk, M.D., et al. NCDAI out of stock
GPO Stock #017-024-00982-2 $6.50 NTIS PB #80-178882 $17.50

30 THEORIES ON DRUG ABUSE: SELECTED CONTEMPORARY PERSPECTIVES. Dan J. Lettieri, Ph.D.; Mollie Sayers; and Helen Wallenstein Pearson, eds. NCDAI out of stock
GPO Stock #017-024-00997-1 $10 Not available from NTIS

31 MARIJUANA RESEARCH FINDINGS: 1980. Robert C. Petersen, Ph.D., ed.
GPO out of stock NTIS PB #80-215171 $20.50

32 GC/MS ASSAYS FOR ABUSED DRUGS IN BODY FLUIDS. Rodger L. Foltz, Ph.D.; Allison F. Fentiman, Jr., Ph.D.; and Ruth B. Foltz.
GPO out of stock NTIS PB #81-133746 $19

33 BENZODIAZEPINES: A REVIEW OF RESEARCH RESULTS, 1980. Stephen I. Szara, M.D., D.Sc., and Jacqueline P. Ludford, M.S., eds.
GPO Stock #017-024-01108-8 $5 NTIS PB #82-139106 $13

34 PROBLEMS OF DRUG DEPENDENCE, 1980: PROCEEDINGS OF THE 42ND ANNUAL SCIENTIFIC MEETING, THE COMMITTEE ON PROBLEMS OF DRUG DEPENDENCE, INC. Louis S. Harris, Ph.D., ed. NCDAI out of stock
GPO out of stock NTIS PB #81-194847 $34

35 DEMOGRAPHIC TRENDS AND DRUG ABUSE, 1980-1995. Louise G. Richards, Ph.D., ed.
GPO out of stock NTIS PB #82-103417 $13

36 NEW APPROACHES TO TREATMENT OF CHRONIC PAIN: A REVIEW OF MULTI-DISCIPLINARY PAIN CLINICS AND PAIN CENTERS. Lorenz K.Y. Ng, M.D., ed.
GPO out of stock NTIS PB #81-240913 $19

37 BEHAVIORAL PHARMACOLOGY OF HUMAN DRUG DEPENDENCE. Travis Thompson, Ph.D., and Chris E. Johanson, Ph.D., eds.
GPO Stock #017-024-01109-6 $7 NTIS PB #82-136961 $25

38 DRUG ABUSE AND THE AMERICAN ADOLESCENT. Dan J. Lettieri, Ph.D., and Jacqueline P. Ludford, M.S., eds.
GPO Stock #017-024-01107-0 $4.50 NTIS PB #82-148198 $14.50

39 YOUNG MEN AND DRUGS IN MANHATTAN: A CAUSAL ANALYSIS. Richard R. Clayton, Ph.D., and Harwin L. Voss, Ph.D.
GPO out of stock NTIS PB #82-147372 $19

40 ADOLESCENT MARIJUANA ABUSERS AND THEIR FAMILIES. Herbert Hendin, M.D., Ann Pollinger, Ph.D., Richard Ulman, Ph.D., and Arthur Carr, Ph.D. NCDAI out of stock
GPO out of stock NTIS PB #82-133117 $13

41 PROBLEMS OF DRUG DEPENDENCE, 1981: PROCEEDINGS OF THE 43RD ANNUAL SCIENTIFIC MEETING, THE COMMITTEE ON PROBLEMS OF DRUG DEPENDENCE, INC. Louis S. Harris, Ph.D., ed. NCDAI out of stock
Not available from GPO NTIS PB #82-190760 $41.50

42 THE ANALYSIS OF CANNABINOIDS IN BIOLOGICAL FLUIDS. Richard L. Hawks, Ph.D., ed.
GPO Stock #017-024-01151-7 $5 NTIS PB #83-136044 $16

43 PROBLEMS OF DRUG DEPENDENCE, 1982: PROCEEDINGS OF THE 44TH ANNUAL SCIENTIFIC MEETING, THE COMMITTEE ON PROBLEMS OF DRUG DEPENDENCE, INC. Louis S. Harris, Ph.D., ed. NCDAI out of stock
GPO out of stock NTIS PB #83-252-692/AS $40

44 MARIJUANA EFFECTS ON THE ENDOCRINE AND REPRODUCTIVE SYSTEMS. Monique C. Braude, Ph.D., and Jacqueline P. Ludford, M.S., eds.
GPO Stock #017-024-01202-5 $4 NTIS PB #85-150563/AS $14.50

45 CONTEMPORARY RESEARCH IN PAIN AND ANALGESIA, 1983. Roger M. Brown, Ph.D.; Theodore M. Pinkert, M.D., J.D.; and Jacqueline P. Ludford, M.S., eds.
GPO Stock #017-024-01191-6 $2.75 NTIS PB #84-184670/AS $11.50

46 BEHAVIORAL INTERVENTION TECHNIQUES IN DRUG ABUSE TREATMENT. John Grabowski, Ph.D.; Maxine L. Stitzer, Ph.D., and Jack E. Henningfield, Ph.D., eds.
GPO Stock #017-024-01192-4 $4.25 NTIS PB #84-184688/AS $16

47 PREVENTING ADOLESCENT DRUG ABUSE: INTERVENTION STRATEGIES. Thomas J. Glynn, Ph.D.; Carl G. Leukefeld, D.S.W.; and Jacqueline P. Ludford, M.S., eds.
GPO Stock #017-024-01180-1 $5.50 NTIS PB #85-159663/AS $22

48 MEASUREMENT IN THE ANALYSIS AND TREATMENT OF SMOKING BEHAVIOR. John Grabowski, Ph.D., and Catherine S. Bell, M.S., eds.
GPO Stock #017-024-01181-9 $4.50 NTIS PB 84-145184 $14.50

49 PROBLEMS OF DRUG DEPENDENCE, 1983: PROCEEDINGS OF THE 45TH ANNUAL SCIENTIFIC MEETING, THE COMMITTEE ON PROBLEMS OF DRUG DEPENDENCE, INC. Louis S. Harris, Ph.D., ed.
GPO Stock #017-024-01198-3 $12 NTIS PB 85-151553/AS $22

50 COCAINE: PHARMACOLOGY, EFFECTS, AND TREATMENT OF ABUSE. John Grabowski, Ph.D., ed.
GPO Stock #017-020-01214-9 $4 NTIS PB 85-150381/AS $14.50

51 DRUG ABUSE TREATMENT EVALUATION: STRATEGIES, PROGRESS, AND PROSPECTS. Frank M. Tims, Ph.D., ed. NCDAI out of stock
GPO Stock #017-020-01218-1 $4.50 NTIS PB 85-150365/AS $17.50

52 TESTING DRUGS FOR PHYSICAL DEPENDENCE POTENTIAL AND ABUSE LIABILITY. Joseph V. Brady, Ph.D., and Scott E. Lukas, Ph.D., eds.
GPO Stock #017-024-01204-1 $4.25 NTIS PB 85-150373/AS $16

54 MECHANISMS OF TOLERANCE AND DEPENDENCE. Charles Wm. Sharp, Ph.D., ed.
GPO Stock #017-024-01213-1 $8.50

55 PROBLEMS OF DRUG DEPENDENCE, 1984. PROCEEDINGS OF THE 46TH ANNUAL SCIENTIFIC MEETING, THE COMMITTEE ON PROBLEMS OF DRUG DEPENDENCE, INC. Louis S. Harris, Ph.D., ed.
GPO Stock #017-024-01242-4 $9.50

56 ETIOLOGY OF DRUG ABUSE: IMPLICATIONS FOR PREVENTION. Coryl LaRue Jones, Ph.D., and Robert J. Battjes, D.S.W., eds.
GPO Stock #017-024-01250-5 $6.50

57 SELF-REPORT METHODS OF ESTIMATING DRUG USE: MEETING CURRENT CHALLENGES TO VALIDITY. Beatrice A. Rouse, Ph.D., Nicholas J. Kozel, M.S., and Louise G. Richards, Ph.D., eds.
GPO Stock #017-024-01246-7 $4.25

58 PROGRESS IN THE DEVELOPMENT OF COST-EFFECTIVE TREATMENT FOR DRUG ABUSERS. Rebecca S. Ashery, D.S.W., ed.
GPO Stock #017-024-01247-5 $4.25

59 CURRENT RESEARCH ON THE CONSEQUENCES OF MATERNAL DRUG ABUSE. Theodore M. Pinkert, M.D., J.D., ed.
GPO Stock #017-024-01249-1 $2.50

60 PRENATAL DRUG EXPOSURE: KINETICS AND DYNAMICS. C. Nora Chiang, Ph.D., and Charles C. Lee, Ph.D., eds.

IN PRESS

53 PHARMACOLOGICAL ADJUNCTS IN SMOKING CESSATION. John Grabowski, Ph.D., ed.

61 COCAINE USE IN AMERICA: EPIDEMIOLOGIC AND CLINICAL PERSPECTIVES. Nicholas J. Kozel, M.S., and Edgar H. Adams, M.S., eds.

62 THE NEUROSCIENCE OF DRUG ABUSE. Roger M Brown, Ph.D., and David P. Friedman, Ph.D., eds.

63 PREVENTION RESEARCH: DETERRING DRUG ABUSE AMONG CHILDREN AND ADOLESCENTS. Catherine S. Bell, M.S.; and Robert J. Battjes, D.S.W., eds.

U.S. GOVERNMENT PRINTING OFFICE : 1985 O - 483-942 : QL 3

DATE DUE

APR 28 1988	APR 29 1988		
OCT 23 1998	OCT 23 1998		

GAYLORD PRINTED IN U.S.A.